inbound

For information, address
Charlotte Martinkus
onetimeiblog@gmail.com

ISBN: 978-0-578-90232-6

Editors:
Lauren Riebs
Sai Leigh

Cover & Interior Design:
Charlotte Martinkus

✕ ✕ ✕

To Mom, Dad, and Phil
for sticking with me even through the times
I blew a gasket.
Love you all, and I'm so excited
for what lies ahead.

✕ ✕ ✕

for my family

There was this warm breeze
and every time I inhaled it,
I inhaled blissful spring mornings in the green grass and
glistening sunlight.
I inhaled patio lunches with my family
and afternoons quietly reading entire compilations of
cartoons in the backyard
while my dad cooks brats on the grill.
I breathed in games of cherry bomb in the park with my
brother, our neighbors,
and Saturday morning car rides to my piano lessons
listening to NPR;
I breathed in chats about nothing and everything with my
mom,
chasing the sun as it sunk into the ground.
My lungs filled with memories of being enveloped by still
wintry Swedish forests,
salty Italian seaside vistas with pearly white homes
blooming from the cliff sides,
walks alongside the Mississippi River laughing with
friends,
and bike rides overlooking Lake Michigan surged through
them.
I breathed the smell of my childhood,
the bittersweetness of growing up,
and leaving those memories behind.
I inhale the warm wind,
the nostalgia for what once was, but
once I exhale, I am at peace
knowing I am making room
for new memories to nourish my lungs
the next time I inhale.

directions

disclaimer

This story focuses on my own recovery and experiences with anxiety, depression, and eating disorders. If you believe this information may be triggering, please either stop here or make sure you have support available while you read.

I would also like to add that though this is a story of my particular demons, I know everyone struggles with demons of varying size and flavor. I realize that I come from a background of privilege, and as such, I can only discuss these issues through my lens as a white, cisgender, heterosexual, middle-class woman. Please read ahead with this in mind.

My story also speaks of sexuality, gender, and sexual harassment. I can only speak from what I know as a cis-heterosexual woman, so while I assume a cis-heterosexual female perspective of gender and sexuality in my writing or poetry, I also recognize that assault and abuse is relevant for all genders and sexual orientations alike, with some being at higher risk than others. The pressures from the institutions upholding the patriarchy have fucked up anybody and everybody, regardless of gender.

home

I used to say I was from Chicago, which was significantly easier than saying Highland Park, a small town in the suburbs just outside the city.

"Oh, so you're not *really* from Chicago," was a common response from people with a verifiable Chicago address, paired with an expression of utmost pride for their own house's geographical location.

In my defense, no one outside of the area knows of Highland Park. Besides, I had family living all over the city, woven through so many different neighborhoods and suburbs from the outskirts to the center that it often felt like I lived in at least a dozen different zip codes. Even as an adult, no matter where in the world I actually live, I always consider this amalgamation of both Chicago's suburbs and its heart my home.

But that's a little complicated. By way of introduction, I would just say I'm from Chicago. (Now I actually live in the city, so no one can tell me otherwise.)

Over the years, I drove my car a fair share throughout the city and the surrounding suburbs. Prior to renting my first apartment in Chicago, I was commuting from my parents' home to the city several days a week in my super adorable but definitely well-used Honda Fit. On a good day, it was only a forty-minute drive.

Most days were not good days.

While driving down I-94, either to class or to goof off with my boyfriend, I usually ended up in rush hour, where it could take anywhere from an hour to two before I finally made it to my destination. I'm sort of getting furious anxiety just thinking about that drive again.

By that point I had driven to and from the city enough times to memorize exit names and their locations in relation to each other. I knew it so well that I would calculate how much farther I had to drive based on which exit sign I saw next. Some exits would bring welcome relief, where traffic almost always flowed smoother, while others provoked absurd fury because I'd realize I was not moving as fast as I normally would. Each exit became a benchmark, relating how far along I was and how much farther I had left to go. At the end of the day I always got there. Perhaps I arrived in various emotional and physical states, depending on how bad traffic was, but I would make it to the city nonetheless.

I sincerely believe life is about the journey rather than the destination, but when that journey gets intense (or rage-inducing like I-94), it helps to have mile markers that represent just how far I've come, and how close I am to where I want to be.

To get through some of the toughest challenges I have faced in my life, I used benchmarks to give me hope and measure my personal growth, just as I do when I'm crawling on the expressway, heading into the city.

This is the story of the progress I've made conquering my demons over the last twenty-eight years, told through both prose and poetry. Whether your struggles mirror mine or diverge completely, I hope you will see yourself in this story and continue to reach toward the benchmarks on your own expressway.

half day road, exit 21

If you played near the end of the piano recital, it meant you were one of the instructor's more advanced students. This was both a great honor and a great burden for me. Each recital suddenly became a terrible waiting game of impending doom.

Though the petrifying fear would always begin months before, the real panic would set in the moment we arrived at the community center. It was a beautiful brick building, as if it might have been a church in its past life. The room of the recital would change from one year to the next, but on performance night, it always looked the same: two grand pianos on one side and a long table filled with treats and lemonade on the other. Just looking at those stacks of cookies toppling onto plates of gooey brownies and chocolate covered pretzels made me queasy; I knew I would only get them if I survived the torture of playing music for fifty random strangers.

As the clock ticked on, I would feel my pulse throbbing throughout my entire body as my lungs weakened. Tears barricaded themselves behind my eyes, preparing for the moment I would inevitably fumble the music or miss a key, ready to unleash themselves in despair. As I waited for my turn, the panic would steadily climb. When it was finally my turn, I would usually play well, as more advanced students should play. The audience would applaud, and I would stumble in a daze back to my seat. For that one moment I could melt into bliss; it was over.

But it would never get easier, despite what my teachers promised. From the age of eight to the time I left for college, I participated in twenty recitals. Every single one felt like my last day to live on earth before being drafted to Satan's army. Whenever I played a song that required the foot pedals, I remember my foot levitating over the suspension pedal, shaking so badly that it both visibly and audibly rumbled the entire grand piano.

Don't get me wrong—performance anxiety is totally normal, but even at a young age I could tell that what I was feeling wasn't. Thinking about the moment at recitals right before I push my fingers down on a set of piano keys still terrifies me to this day.

At the time, my family and I just thought I was kind of batshit crazy (and to be fair, we still sometimes feel that way). I would have crying spells out of nowhere or be unable to handle to-do lists with more than one item on them. This, we thought, was simply my personality. I was fortunate enough to lead a lovely childhood with caring people, a safe environment, and financial stability. What could possibly be wrong with me?

Later when I was in my early twenties we learned that my doctor had diagnosed me with Generalized Anxiety Disorder when I was very young. Somehow, she neglected to tell me or my family about it at the time. For years we remained unaware of any reason for my panic or anxiety. We just assumed it must not be a problem.

But, of course, it was. And it was really fucking confusing.

✕ ✕ ✕

my heart is on the track team without me

My pulse begins to race
first the fifty-meter dash
then the hundred
four hundred
eight hundred
the mile
it keeps going, racing

no end, no reward
except a proud coach: my hungry anxiety.
no participation prize,
just a pleased expression from its face,
reaping my awards as its own.

Still my heart sprints,
sometimes in a relay with my lungs,
my breath shortens
as the race lengthens
until anxiety
loosens the reins on my pulse
and allows it to finally
pace itself.

✕ ✕ ✕

As young as five years old, I was acutely aware
of how others perceived me. By meticulously watching

the way others interacted I concluded that I didn't quite fit within the context of many social situations. I would constantly fear saying the wrong thing, hurting someone's feelings, or making the wrong impression. I couldn't even read, yet I could worry about my social impact.

But I did think like that. I grew up thinking that my emotions, needs, wants—none of it mattered because if I thought about any of those things, I was selfish.

I was also becoming extremely sensitive to how people around me were feeling at any given moment. When my brother carelessly broke his retainer as a kid, I offered to personally pay for it because I didn't want my family to bear the burden. I was nine years old; there's no way I could have afforded that. Regardless, I felt this deep remorse and responsibility to resolve the problem and I would dwell on it for days.

Without any influence from my friends or family, I put extreme amounts of pressure on myself to be perfect. My grades, behaviors, relationships, piano playing—even when I practiced alone—all needed to be no less than exemplary at every moment. Being naturally ambitious only exacerbated the high standards my anxiety placed on me. Even the smallest trigger would send me spiraling me into a panic that I felt unable to express or describe to anyone around me.

So when I said something embarrassing in front of my cousins when I was four? Panic attack.

When I didn't think I was cool enough to pull off Converse when I was six? Panic attack.

When I felt overwhelmed at school when my mom was away at work when I was seven? Panic attack.

When I was given more than one homework assignment when I was nine? Panic attack.

When I got a three out of four on a quiz when I was twelve? Panic attack.

13

When I failed an exam when I was fifteen and I thought I would never surmount to anything? Major panic attack.

Welcome to my anxiety.

✕ ✕ ✕

the outcast

I am the outcast,
the third wheel
willing to walk
on the grass, in the street,
scrape against the bushes
so that the rest of the group stays in tune,
safe from the world around them
on the paved path they travel.

I am the outcast,
the freak.
I speak in tones
and think in colors
I try to morph, shape-shift
to look like a triangle
or square or trapezoid
but I will only ever be
an unusual shape
with undefined angles
that no one can name.

I am the outcast,
the mute mime
dancing only in shadows

and hidden corners—
isolated, off stage
so the rest of the dancers
can maintain their predetermined rhythm
without needing to match mine.

I am the outcast
it is my feet that step outside the boundary
it is my hands that put on the mask
that says I'm lesser, different
telling the world that
I am not a part of it.

The only reason I am the outcast
is because I call myself one.

ego

I admire those who are different than me
but I punish myself for being different than them.

What is acceptable for them
is not acceptable for me.

When did I become so arrogant
to believe I am so goddamn special?

That if they are one way
I must be better?

When did my ego inflate so large
that it left no room for being human?

orbits

I take an elliptical orbit,
while many others move in perfect circles
but we all still orbit a burning sun.

I was given life by the same dying stars,
my bones crackle with stardust and so do yours;
How can any one of us be otherly
when at the core we are the same?

flicker

I flicker like a star
except instead of a sphere of flame and gas
I am a swirling sphere of

that feeling
when my heart thuds so hard
that it begins to erode the walls
of my chest, and yet,
I am incapacitated under blankets, alone,
because even opening my eyes
requires the strength to bend steel

that feeling
when I'm invincible,
keeping dry while in the midst of a thunderstorm, and yet,
that smudge on the middle of the window
that can't be wiped away
as hard as you damn try

because it's on the other side
of the glass

that feeling
when the sun strokes my skin
on a bath of sand, and yet,
a typhoon explodes from my eyes
because I am a natural disaster
that can sneak up any time of day
with no warning nor reason

that feeling
when chaos and logic
coexist on the same plane
in neither one nor the other
in all that, I flicker.

It no longer surprises me
that stars don't simply disappear
when they die—

they erupt.

deerfield road, exit 24

I refused to wear dresses starting in first grade. Even in my six-year-old brain, I knew dresses were considered feminine and being feminine was considered weak. Every time I put one on, whether for a ballet recital or a formal occasion, my heart rate blew to smithereens. Even though I've always been surrounded by powerful and independent women—and those role models have been crucial—I've also always struggled with my womanhood and female body. Having chronic anxiety only exacerbated the way I responded to those struggles. Instead of ignoring them like normal six-year-olds, my anxiety's reaction to my uncertain but very big feelings was deciding that dresses could no longer be a part of my wardrobe.

This is the first rebellion I can remember against my female form. It was from then on that I fought valiantly to reject expressing my assigned gender because I saw it as a flaw, a weakness. I saw it as something that would hinder my future success and the way I was respected within the world.

I remember playing flag football once in elementary school and the team had me act as the quarterback because the teacher told the boys they needed to do a better job including the girls. Tossing around a football happens to be something I genuinely enjoy, so just as I did with my dad and brother at home, I threw a beautiful spiral exactly where it needed to go. The boys gazed at me, shocked, unable to believe I could possess such a skill. Tossing that ball even better than most of the boys had me brimming with power, because suddenly I wasn't just a girl, but a valuable girl because I had masculine skills.

These traits could only get me so far, however. I realized that the media, and therefore the rest of society, idolize women of beauty. A woman didn't necessarily have to be good at sports to be respected, as long as she possessed undeniable beauty. And beauty, I quickly learned, was thinness.

Women, from what I noticed, craved thin waists. As young as nine years old, I would receive compliments from people about my thin figure, as if it was this wonderful thing. My body seemed to evoke jealousy, adoration, even acceptance from other people—so much so that I actually started to believe it. I started to realize the advantages, the admiration, that came along with my thinness.

But at this point the process of hiding my femininity to exaggerate any masculine traits I might have was second nature—I did it without even thinking. If I could simultaneously have this beauty piece, this thinness desired in women, and masculine skills, I realized I could be invincible. How could I be bullied, how could I be an outcast, how could I be disliked if I possessed those traits most desired in humans?

So I stopped wearing dresses. My favorite colors changed from pink and purple to green. I continued to tweak seemingly trivial things about myself with the hope that I wouldn't solely be seen as a girl, but a valuable girl. I ingrained this within myself so deeply that whenever I wrote stories growing up, I usually pictured the main character as a boy. To this day, sometimes my inner voice is a man. I clung to any masculine personality traits I had in the hope that they would keep me safe from ridicule and protect me from the inevitable weakness I believed I inherited from simply existing as a girl. I think this is when I first saw my eating disorder (ED) in passing, without even realizing what that meant.

✕✕✕

synonyms

People would always say to me,
"You're so beautiful—,
You're so thin,"
so often that
in my mind,
beautiful and thin
became synonyms.

charlotte, meet ED

The first time I realized
my body was unacceptable
was in fifth grade.
My widening hips,
my rounding stomach
should have been indications
that I was taking on
one of earth's most exquisite forms:

a woman.

Instead I saw
a widening crevice
cracking open,
separating me
from thinness,
from beauty.

And I remember explicitly
for a moment,
my panic was slightly abated
when I noticed
I was still
the thinnest girl in my class.

✗ ✗ ✗

Of course, I could not tuck away my femininity forever. Puberty came knocking and whooped my ass. (Does anyone, to be fair, actually have a wonderful, simple time with puberty?) Where I once thought I only had to worry about whether or not I should wear dresses, puberty threw a new card into the ring: sex.

When I first got my period, I felt so much shame. I cried. Sobbed, rather. I didn't want to be a woman. I didn't want boobs or a period or a vagina. I definitely didn't want to have sex. I rejected sexuality completely. Like my gender, I thought sexuality made me a weak and morally tainted person. Most teens get embarrassed around their crushes and budding romances, but I made it an extreme sport.

Every school dance or Bar/Bat Mitzvah party (of which I went to a surprising number for a Catholic girl) became a high-level game of hide-and-seek. These events were already dangerous territory because they required wearing dresses, applying makeup, and straightening our hair. My mom would fuss over me, helping me with an outfit and doing my hair. She was adorable and sweet, but I doubt she remembers these moments fondly; I always put up a huge tantrum. I didn't want my hair, face, or body to resemble that of a woman's. I didn't want to wear a dress that accentuated my curves and attracted all the boys. I wanted to hide my body and become an amorphous blob that could dance with my friends in peace.

But then the slow songs would start to play. My heart would hammer through my chest and I would bolt to the bathroom or the refreshments table. I wanted to be physically unable to participate. I had a lot of success with this method—until one middle school dance when a very cute boy completely took me by surprise. I was eating snacks at a table, normally a safe haven, when he thwarted my plan by asking me to dance. Terrified, the food I had just munched down almost came right back up again. The sensation of my pulse thumped louder than the music in our school auditorium. The thought of touching his shoulders, his hands upon my waist, even innocently, sent me reeling. Paralyzed, I outright told him no and ran to the bathroom, now my only respite. I left him standing there while guilt bubbled inside me.

During this time, I became very familiar with the hotel bathrooms across the Chicago area—and I can tell you that this city has some fine restroom facilities.

✕ ✕ ✕

asleep

I always thought ED was dormant for the early years of
my life
when in reality
he was feasting on the warped ideas I soaked up
until he could grow strong enough to overtake me.

turning tables

Whenever I would hear
girls fret about their new diet,
the treats they craved that were off-limits,
the meals they yearned for that were an absolute "No,"
so they could
fit into that dress, sculpt themselves
in order to dazzle in their new bikini,

I would roll my eyes,
finish my bag of cookies,
or burger with fries,
with a non-diet soda or two;
my three meals a day
and wonder what it must be like
to be terrorized by that which nourishes them.

Now here I am.

lake cook road, exit 25A

It was five in the morning and I still hadn't gone to bed. I was sitting in my college dorm, working through my physics homework and still had several unfinished, unanswered problems remaining. No matter how long I stared at the equations, the mysterious concoctions of Greek letters wrapped up in calculus, I didn't know how to solve them. What I did know was that if I went to bed without finishing my homework, I would be a failure.

I sat in my apartment questioning why I studied physics, why I was at this school, and why I was so stupid that I couldn't figure out electromagnetism. I resisted calling home all night until finally I just couldn't handle it; I needed help. My dad would probably be getting ready for work, or maybe already be on the train, so I decided to call him first. Despite the early hour of the long day ahead of him, he answered. With his calm, even voice, he talked me through my panic until it subsided.

My college years were full of times like this. Under the pressure of higher education, the intensity of my anxiety grew without bounds. Everything I worried about as a kid suddenly became real: I was no longer achieving good grades, no longer surrounded by friends, and no longer had any confidence in my intellect. My parents had invested a huge sum of money into my education and therefore my future, and yet I felt like an idiot with no academic or personal prospects.

My social life wasn't much better. I was struggling to make many friends in or outside of my major. When people did invite me to hang out, I often refused because I was always catching up on homework or exhausted from the work I'd already done. I longed to have a normal college experience, but I felt like an outlier among my social circles.

The only thing I had under control was my looks. I was considered pretty, and by pretty, I mean thin. As long as I stayed thin, it didn't matter if I was incompetent or lonely because I would still have worth. The "Freshman Fifteen" loomed over me, and I became hyper-aware of my eating habits. Thinness was the last branch I held onto; if it broke, I was sure that I would fall into a chasm of bottomless failure. Or something to that effect.

As my anxieties continued to mount, I abandoned piano and photography to focus on surviving classes and self-loathing. When I needed a break, I went to parties where I found I could self-medicate my anxiety and stress with the numbing effects of alcohol. I never became addicted, but I did abuse it.

With little sleep and an empty stomach, I would black out most nights I drank. I would wake up the next morning in an even more troubled emotional state than the day before, shamed that I drank so much, but that never negated the fact that in the moment of abyss, the numbness was absolutely beautiful.

✕ ✕ ✕

when I need a break

The alcohol runs its shimmering tendrils over my mind
through dark canals,
hopping across bridges between neurons
in search of peace, inner peace,
just a piece
to toss to my anxiety,
a ravenous beast untamed.

As it seeks,
anxiety traces the spectacle, distracted,
and peace appears for just a moment
a dandelion feather about to vanish in the sky
but alcohol is blind, and alcohol is determined
and though peace is fluttering above, alcohol starts to
settle in,
first brushing off shallow worries gathering dust
then moving on to insecurities—
those pulsing, unwavering,
very much alive and very much despised—
they resurface.

The beast howls
choking on the smoke of emerging emotion
and here alcohol leaves me,
both of us defeated.
But oh, the messy bundle it turns me into
is worth uprooting that pain, and all the vacancies left
behind,
to try and catch that fleeting dandelion feather
to hold it in my hand just once
to smell its sweet earth
and think of nothing else.

X X X

I thought I was just "a little stressed out." Everyone at my school was, right? It would have been too embarrassing for me to talk to my brilliant, incredible professors about how I was struggling, so I kept it to myself. My close friends and family probably had their suspicions, but no one knew how to address it. Hell, I didn't even know what was happening. I just found myself in these heightened states of panic from which I couldn't come down.

Living on my own, and without my parents around to help bring me down, I turned to more dangerous vices at my disposal. While alcohol was a major coping mechanism available to me, it was not the only one.

The other major vice was food.

Around this time in my life I studied abroad, which more often than not became eating abroad. With every *kanelbullar* and glass of pear cider, I was losing some of the thinness I had come to rely on. Paired with a strong anxiety disorder and newly developing depression, an eating disorder (often dubbed ED) was officially born.

My minor weight gain wasn't catastrophic strictly because I needed slightly larger pants. It was catastrophic to me because it meant I lacked the discipline to control my weight, the one thing I had left in my control. I was officially a failure and the one "good" thing about me had vanished. And yes, eating disorders are about losing weight and being thin, but for me, it was more about proving to myself that I was both in control and valuable. Even if I couldn't control my grades, friends, or life in general, at least I would be able to control this.

This type of thinking and behavior became an addiction. I couldn't stop starving myself. I felt compelled to exercise constantly, multiple times a day if I didn't have class. I counted every calorie. I linked my self-worth inextricably with my anorexic and orthorexic (and later binge-eating and bulimic) behaviors.

The anxiety reached a level where I would rather not be conscious in my own life. This starvation cycle gave me a sort of high to cope through it. Without proper nutrients, the brain can't function normally and has to reallocate resources. During those starvation periods, it became impossible to think straight. All I could hear was a loud voice in my head, cheering me on for my impressive control, for refusing to eat as much as my body actually needed. In this clouded delirium, I felt like hot shit.

The eating disorder voice in my mind, one I would soon become very familiar with, celebrated my absolute genius. Everything else was kept at bay when I was riding this high. But inevitably, I'd need to eat at some point, and the whole beautiful mirage would crumble.

✕ ✕ ✕

letter to my body #1: attack

Of all the hands, all the feet
all the arms, legs, faces, waists
I am stuck with you.
Trapped
my only way to interact with the world
is through you.
I smell through your lumpy nose
touch with your stubby, cracked fingers
taste through your mustached lips and dopey smile.
You isolate me

from the gorgeous girls around me
sprinkling zits on your plain face
and teasing your knotted hair
yet nothing is funny
about attempting to squeeze myself into
a box which I will never fit.
Other girls saunter gracefully in elegant clothes
and I am carried by you.
Bulky, gawky, awkward,

average.

Your stomach bulges over your pants as I write this.
Your arm fat jiggles as my pencil scratches the paper.
Your thighs chafe as I shift in my chair.
I need to exert so much effort
to fix you
to try to make you look
like the pretty girl I am inside of you.

But there are only so many outfits
with baggy sweaters
and expandable waistbands
I can wear to hide in shame
for I must be seen
through you.

set theory

{brave, creative, independent, genuine, determined, witty, driven, adventurous, amiable, bright, thin, pretty}

{brave, independent, genuine, determined, driven, amiable, bright, thin, pretty}

{brave, independent, determined, driven, bright, thin, pretty}

{independent, driven, bright, thin, pretty}

{bright, thin, pretty}

{thin, pretty}

{ }

{anxiety}

{anxiety, depression}

{anxiety, depression, insecurity}

{anxiety, depression, insecurity, turbulence}

{anxiety, depression, insecurity, turbulence, unraveling}

{anxiety, depression, insecurity, turbulence, unraveling, eating disorder}

tower road, exit 31

As I slid deeper into my addiction, I began to crave new avenues of validation. I had long resented my assigned gender and now resented my body, but it seemed the men of the world felt differently. Strangers would hit on me all the time, whether at the bar or on the street. In a way this felt normal; I had the stereotypical "hot girl" body, which to me meant I was a pair of tits worth their attention. It didn't matter to me that these men didn't get to know me or even my name. I determined, whether true or not, that my personality was irrelevant, as long as my body was desired. I processed everything through the context of my own body insecurity. Maybe some guys did want to meet me for my personality but at the time, I was wearing my anxiety and ED glasses. The only reality I could see was that men wanted me for my appearance alone.

This was the message reinforced to me over and over again. My friends and I had been inappropriately approached or touched so many times, I could list examples for days. Once, a guy grabbed a hunk of my butt while I was waiting at a bus stop. Ask any woman—I'm sure they'll be thrilled to tell you about their own tales.

So throughout college, femininity was all physical. As one of the few female physics majors, I felt that in order to hold my own and be respected amongst my male peers I needed to either abandon my femininity or be overtly feminine in a sexual way. There was this looming bro culture, and these were the only ways I felt I could penetrate it. To be clear, nobody ever told me this explicitly; all of my male peers were supportive and kind. Yet, I was constantly aware of the fact that I was a woman surrounded by men.

Part of the problem was that I looked to the boys around me to validate me as a person. If these men I highly respected flirted with me, maybe I could one day be respected too. Nothing ever went beyond flirting, so I ended up drunkenly searching for self-respect in the mouths of random guys. (Spoiler alert: I never found it there.)

Around this time, I began letting guys make out with me. It was something I thought I owed to my partners because they gave me the companionship and attention I craved. Everything was a tradeoff, an exchange of goods. However, while we were physically in the same room, my mind would always be elsewhere, dissociated from my body. In my head, I would tell myself jokes, make to-do lists for the next day, perform an exhaustive analysis on whatever music that was playing. One time, I did some rehab exercises for my recently torn ankle while some poor guy was trying to kiss me. Even the very first time I kissed a boy, I was planning out my essay on the Hmong sudden unexplained nocturnal death syndrome. I think I actually made some progress that night. With the paper, I mean. It didn't matter to me that my mind wandered or that I didn't enjoy myself because I felt I was giving boys the only part of me that was valuable: my body in return for their affection.

When people sustain trauma or mental illness, regardless of what those may be, one of the common responses can be to separate oneself from one's reality, because reality is where that trauma lives. Alcohol and drugs became tools that helped with this body-mind separation, as they do for many others as well. I didn't want to deal with the anxiety of connecting my body, this tangible bridge to reality, to the concepts of femininity and sexuality, so I literally tried to separate myself in any way I could: I withdrew into my mind. The more I retreated into my mind, the more resentful I became of my body; after all, my body was the reason I felt the edge of my anxiety, the weight of my depression, the hunger of my eating disorder.

✕ ✕ ✕

no wonder

Shamed are women who give too little.
Shamed are women who give too much.
Shamed are men who take too little.
Glorified are men who take too much.

Yet somehow
many still wonder
as to what kind of chain
slaves away
on rape culture—
a culture of taking
and never giving—
motorizing it, mobilizing it,
empowering it
to thrive.

no

You can say no
even though he wants a yes.
Rights should not be distributed
according to sex organs.
Rights are as natural as rain is wet.
When he thrusts his opinions
about your shape, your ass
into your ear;
when his gaze clasps tightly to your breasts
when his hands anchor themselves to your ass;
when he tries to carve his number into your skin
while burning your neck with his kisses,
melding his crotch into yours,
because he thinks he's doing you a favor
say It with so much power
the sun is jealous.
No.

violation

What he did to you
what he took of yours
what he touched
with his fingers
with his lips
makes me want to rip away
all their fingers, all their lips
because I know of no other way
to protect you.

the world we live in

I think about all the times
I would have been assaulted
I was careless
I let my guard down
I gave my trust too easily
but I never was assaulted
because I was lucky.
Isn't it sad
that I am grateful for the times
my body wasn't violated?
Isn't it sad
that the power to violate my body
lies entirely in I's and me's,
my hands, my voice?
Isn't it sad
that if I don't keep a watchful eye
then I feel I deserved it?

vocalizing

He speaks of his anger, so I look down
the words fall apart in my throat
and cascade into my belly.
I revel in the power he has
to crack every sentence I try to create
to shatter the opinions that attempt to assemble

I admire the women who still manage to make a sound
in spite of the gag he shoves in their mouths.

don't tell me I'm beautiful

Don't tell me I'm beautiful
with your lips.
Say it with your eyes
as you lie on my thighs,
don't lie
like the others,
silky sweet
adjectives bubbling from their mouths
a geyser, old faithful,
yet only faithful to my curves
a hot spring about to erupt
but desiring only the syrupy magma
in my blood to make it gush.

Don't tell me I'm beautiful
with viscous words dripping
off your tongue
like the others,
capturing me
with their carefully arranged alphabet
betting I want to be their solution
they lust for me as a catalyst,
waiting for a reaction
that will never commence,
not because I am noble
but because
their seemingly basic letters
are the acid that burns me.

Don't tell me I'm beautiful
with vocal cords
vibrating like the others,

show me
with the pads of your fingers,
uncertain as they meet my skin, timid,
intimidated to touch something so precious
they wear me, aware of their overwhelming addiction
to the way I remove you from our reality
as we become invisible to everything.

Don't tell me I'm beautiful
like the others,
look at me
like you think I'm crazy
so I know you're crazy about me.
Replace the emptiness of words
with the fullness of gesture
because words are plastic
that cracks when I inevitably disagree
whereas gestures never lie
so lie next to me and
don't tell me I'm beautiful;
show me.

my ladies

I only feel weak
because the women I surround myself with
are so strong.

I am only strong
because the women I surround myself with
are so fierce.

willow road, exit 33B

The first time I considered therapy was when some of my close friends were struggling through their own crises and I sought a professional to better understand how I could support them. I toyed with the idea for weeks until I finally booked an appointment with the school therapist.

The office was in the same building as the workout facilities, so I had to walk in my street clothes through the building full of sweaty, athletic college students, practically declaring to all of them that I was going to therapy. Even though I was only there to talk about my friends, I felt extremely nervous. I sat down in the small, warmly lit office, and he asked me what I wanted to talk about. I told him about my friends, and he listened without judgement; I could tell he was on my side and wanted to help.

When I left, I was feeling better, armed with new information to help my friends. Yet I still felt lost because I couldn't solve their problems, and neither could he. Nobody could.

I visited a couple times and each time I felt this burning desire to talk about myself and the chaos manifesting in my own brain, but part of me had convinced myself that it would be selfish—my friends needed the help, not me. At this point, I still didn't even consider my problems to be problems at all. I believed that because I was a white heterosexual female from a healthy, middle-class American family, I wasn't allowed to have problems.

Still, when the therapist would ask pointed questions about my friends and their anxieties, a tiny voice in my head would try to speak up and say, "Hey! I have anxieties too!" Each time, I swallowed the words and buried them into nonexistence. It just didn't occur to me that both my friends could be having a rough time *and* I could also be having a rough time. "And" is a powerful word—we really need to use it more often.

It would be a few years later, after graduation, that I would finally seek support for myself. To be honest, it was almost an accident. I was enrolled in an atmospheric physics PhD program at Penn State University and was deeply unhappy. While the work was fascinating and inspired the type of projects I'd like to work on now, being back in school reopened the chest of trauma I thought I'd left behind in my undergraduate years, and I was unsure how to make it better. I decided to speak with a school counselor to ask for their opinion. Seemed innocent enough. Since it was my first visit with the university's health clinic, they requested I fill out an extensive questionnaire about my mental health.

It was then that I first noticed something was off. For nearly every food-related and anxiety question, I responded poorly.

Can you get through the day without worrying about what you will eat? Strongly disagree.

Do you avoid certain foods because they feel unsafe? Strongly agree.

Do you make excuses to eat alone? Strongly agree. Interesting.

In truth, I always had my suspicions. I noticed my anxiety voice often worked in tangent with a more food-obsessed voice. I knew my behaviors resembled those associated with eating disorders. Still, I had a considerably "normal" weight and, let's face it, a fair share of denial.

With this affirmation of what I suspected deep down, along with the fact that one of my close friends was a huge advocate of mental health—and specifically depression medications—I decided to finally see a doctor. My grades were absolute garbage, the thoughts whirling around my brain never stopped screaming at me, and I avoided interacting with people whenever I could. I just didn't have the energy to come up with excuses not to seek help anymore, so I went.

The doctor was astute. Having reviewed my questionnaire results, she began probing me about my relationship with food. I walked away from that appointment with the anti-depression prescription I wanted, but she also insisted I make an appointment with a specialist in eating disorders.

This second doctor sounded a blaring alarm in my brain. Everything she said rang with eerie accuracy. I had never been able to verbalize the chaos and fear mounting inside my head. I was stunned. For the first time, someone was fluent in the language of my personal disorders, and that was a comfort beyond words.

That appointment, that doctor, launched me into my recovery. I knew I had to trust her. That was the first moment I tasted the sweet drops of healing. As scary as it was, it tasted delicious. From then on I slowly began to build my support team—first with professionals, and then close family and friends. It wasn't going to be an easy road ahead and letting in people I loved and trusted was going to be key.

✕ ✕ ✕

(dis)ordered

Disordered is
eating the foods I love
and calling them fear foods
because when I consume them
I star in my very own horror movie.
As my weight grows
my poltergeists tease me, I lose control.
Shame and guilt chase me, weaving, creeping until
I am tired and my lungs ache.
Disappointment comes after me
with a sharp knife
because I shouldn't have eaten that
because it's bad,
evil, cursed and wretched,
but I did.
I head to the door looming at the end of the hallway
while everyone watching screams at me to just keep
walking
and I open it anyway
the fear foods strangle me
I hunger for starvation
but I end up eating more than the day before
I star in the sequel to the movie
curled up in a ring on the floor
painful emotions flowing out of me
through my violent tears
and I don't know how to guide them.
I sometimes crawl to the bathroom

try to exorcise the poison
but it never works
I just keep conjuring more
because I neglected the rules, dismissed the signs
I failed to ignore
all food in the first place
continuing the cycle
twenty-eight days
weeks
years later
all I want is to just get out
escape this twilight zone
deprived of all logic
this food will haunt me
one Friday the thirteenth after another
until it finally occurs to me
that food is just nourishment wearing a grotesque mask
haunting my little world
and the more I let it into my life
the smaller all those monsters will become
only then will these nightmares become memories
wrapped on a film reel
to be dug out only on the most special of
Halloween nights.

tangibility

When I wake up
to see if I deserve to be loved today
I strangle the skin around my hips
and see how much of my
luscious curves

can fit within my fingers;
my body is objectively,
mathematically quantifiable,
easily malleable in the eyes of my disorders
unlike the shards of my soul.

Though these delicate shards do exist
like the soft flesh I always grasp,
I will never be able to perfect them,
polish the pieces until they are so pristine
that the delicate stamp my fingerprints leave
becomes visible
when I hold them up
and watch the light
dance
on their glimmering surfaces.

skokie road, exit 34A

"Are you sure you want to eat that?"

"Obviously," I sigh. "Would I be making toast with peanut butter if I didn't want to eat it?"

"It sounds like you're second guessing yourself," the voice in my head continues. "You haven't forgotten how many calories are in that, have you?"

"Blah, blah, blah—I can't hear you! Maybe I should eat three pieces of toast with peanut butter, just to show you who's boss."

"Three? Well, that'll take a three-hour walk to work off. Are you sure about that?"

Another voice with a similar timbre blurts out, "Don't do it! If I push your heart rate up any higher, you'll have a heart attack! For the love of God, don't do it! I can't take it, I can't take it—"

"See?" he first voice coos. "Just don't do it. Don't eat any of it. It's better for all of us."

"It's just a piece of toast—"

"But if you eat it, you'll go against our plan," the voices sing together. "Don't let a piece of toast stand between you and what you could be. It's just not worth it. You've already worked so hard, come this far."

"Shut the fuck up!"

I shake my head vigorously, hoping the voices will fly out, but it only amplifies them. The only way to stop their incessant berating would be to eat nothing at all or eat everything and purge. Even then, they might only stop for a moment. But what I would give for a moment of internal silence.

It wasn't always this intense. In fact, though voices like Anxiety have been chatting with me as long as I've been alive, I never thought of them as separate entities from myself. When I heard that voice asking if I was really sure everything would be okay and if I was absolutely certain that people enjoyed my company, I simply thought this was the voice of my better judgement wanting to protect me by teaching me this pessimistic skepticism. This voice spoke with friendly and warm tones, trying so hard to keep me safe; why would it be any different than my own?

As I grew older, this voice shifted and multiplied into many. Despite how harsh they became, I still didn't think anything of it. This was just my better judgement; I was simply being realistic. Why should I be wary of my judgement if it had always been looking out for me?

Therapy is where I was first able to turn this internal monologue between me and my judgement into a dialogue between me and these parasitic voices that thought it best for me to live life on their terms. These voices even had names: Anxiety, Depression, Perfectionism, and ED, my eating disorder. As I spoke, my therapist would address the voice directly. "I'm talking to Anxiety right now, aren't I?" or "Is that what you think, or is that what ED is telling you?"

During this time, my whole mentality started to shift; I would play out the speech in my head as if reading the script to a play, where each of us had our own part. Their lines were always commanding, always condescending. They never commemorated or celebrated me. They would always tack a "but…" to the end of my thoughts when I should have been using "and…" Nothing I ever did satiated these voices or their needs, no matter how much I tried to appease them.

Anxiety would tell me that I was a failure, my work was terrible, and that people spent time with me out of pity. It would lecture me on how selfish I was for celebrating myself or giving attention to my needs. Depression was more soothing in its words. It would tuck me into bed in the middle of a bright day and tell me to take a rest, maybe watch TV for hours on end because nothing would ever get better. Perfectionism shared most of its scenes with Anxiety unless I wanted to work on a project, either academic or otherwise. In those moments, I assure you, Perfectionism spouted beautiful monologues so alluring I felt compelled to stop my project and go back to napping with Depression.

ED, however, was on a whole other level, playing off of everyone else. He devised a way to intertwine with any plot twist thrown at him. He even found ways to dominate a scene without any lines, coercing the other voices to reacting a certain way or forcing me to behave differently. He was as dangerous as he was sneaky, disguising himself in such a way that I sometimes found it impossible to tell whether he was with me or not.

Like Anxiety and Depression, ED appeared friendly at first. He would suggest eating fewer cookies or eating sandwiches without bread to limit my carb intake. It didn't actually seem like a bad idea since I had often heard doctors and the media make similar suggestions.

But then ED created more rules that doctors wouldn't suggest or that I had never heard before. One such rule was that I should always be able to see the protrusion of my ribs and spine through my skin. He had a rule for everything. No matter what food I ate or outfit I wore, ED had a reprimand locked and loaded. His voice made me skeptical about my self-worth and especially my relationship with food, but it was at this point I gained special awareness about what that really meant and how he was attacking me apart from the other voices.

✕ ✕ ✕

ticks

I want to rip it out of me,
this selfish parasite,
using my power to fuel its own,
embedding itself into my skin.

Seemingly impossible to remove,
I can't shake it off,
I can't blow it away,
buried in my skin it remains.

Some days I pick up the tweezers,
ready to dig it out
and remove its toxic flesh from mine,
indifferent to the vulnerable wound it would leave behind.

I need to pluck it out, but it's in so deep.
It won't let go.
My tweezers can't reach it,
they only fuel a desperate rush
to extract as much of me as it can
before I finally decide to fight it.

The harder I pull, the harder it grasps
onto me with its tiny claws.
I finally try, put thoughts to action,
pinching the wretched thing
that thinks it knows me,
thinks it controls me,
because it had invaded me
and usurped my life
with its poisonous daggers.

At last, when I think I'm rid of it,
its body squirming powerlessly in my hands,
I realize its head—
its merciless head—
remains under my skin;
sucking, sipping, draining
me of myself.

One day, I will find its head tucked under my skin.
One day, I will find the strength to remove it,
to pry it away from the warmth of my body,
to burn it so that it can never return to me.
But until that day that it drives me.
It controls me from within
and weakens me with its disease.

Until that day when I can escape from its tight grip
I will be it and it will be me.
Until that day we are one in the same,
but on that day, I will be free.

growth and takeover

As I carve
this malignant tumor
from my depths,
I notice
its tissue crawled, attached itself
to my heart,
my brain,
my soul;
if I remove it,
slice the connections
that have grown so thick you would
think
its tendrils were supposed to be there,
what will become of
the spaces left behind?

✕ ✕ ✕

A major benchmark for me once I finally got my-
self into therapy was identifying that as humans we are
built of many moving parts, a concoction of voices in our
minds that dictate what we say, do, and think. We have
so many components to our identity that, when summed
together, make a person. But while I have anxiety, I am not
my anxiety. I can talk back. I can stand up for myself.

In the beginning of my journey, all I could do was
give names to each voice and learn about them. When are
they loudest? What makes them tick? What makes them
excited? I got to know them like someone gets to know a
new friend.

I quickly realized that these voices, these friends

that had taken care of me, protected me in my most stressful moments, were the same voices that were now destroying me. And these voices were not the same as my own; we never read any of the same lines in the script. All my life I thought I had this slightly more aggressive voice of reason, when in reality my Anxiety, Depression, Perfectionism, and ED where the ones judging reality for me. At first, I felt I could no longer trust myself; the ultimate form of betrayal.

This awareness shed light on a fact I ignored for a long time: I did not consider my body to be a part of me. It was a separate being from myself, almost as if it were a shitty apartment my soul was renting until it could afford a better, more extravagant place. The voices signed the lease without me; my body was no longer a shelter for me.

Awareness of this concept has been such a key point in my recovery, a key exit to reach on my expressway. I could start asking myself questions: Why is the Anxiety voice inside me so loud right now? Why does ED keep talking about my stomach? Why does Perfectionism show up whenever I try to be creative? Why won't Depression let me go out with my friends? They have no ground to stand on, no evidence supporting that they're right. But they are loud as hell.

I then began to recognize them as voices unique from my own true voice. So when I heard a thought, if I identified it as one of these dangerous voices, I could begin to challenge the thought. Eventually I learned not only to challenge it, but to actually act against that thought to the point where many of my behaviors no longer existed. Little by little, an actual voice of reason began to bloom in my mind. Little by little, I began to trust myself again.

✕ ✕ ✕

why I anthropomorphize my eating disorder

I thought it was a part of me,
like
my little pinky toes or
the flecks
of copper floating in my cerulean eyes.
It came as naturally as laughter
or the way
my eyelashes stick together when I cry.
I thought it was an echo
of my own voice
its needs were my needs,
its cravings
were my cravings
when it wanted to punish me
it was a reflection of the consequences
I believed I deserved.

There was no it and me;
only we.
Only us.
But then I turned around
and realized
the shadow at my feet, which
had crept
behind me all these years
looked nothing like me.
The rules and
the voice
that cracked
a whip at my self-worth—
so brutal
the pain still reverberates through

my nervous system,
the blood still crawls
down my skin;
a detached entity.

It glommed itself to me
and I never noticed
enough to distinguish a difference.
Though its fingers grew deep into my psyche
and its cells looked like my own,
its DNA
differed from mine.
I could peel it away
the tunnels it dug through me could close
and I would be left
with myself,
a shadow whose arms would
stretch
toward the sky like mine,
whose hair
would dance in the breeze like mine,
completely,
one hundred percent,
me.
The hardest step was accepting
it had nourished me with propaganda
for all these years.

The hardest step was accepting
we
was really
it
plus
me.

if ED just abandons me here

When he carelessly tosses
all of my pain, all of my symptoms
in his bag and
stomps out the door
I run,
fast and desperate, I try to catch up,
I beckon to him,
shivering because I was too rushed
to find my coat
or my shoes;

dirty twigs prick my bare feet
but none of it matters if he doesn't hear me,
my house is so empty without him there
without his clutter,
without his loud, commanding voice
filling every room
so there is almost no longer
space for me
but I call to him
as he hurls his bag into the taxi,
I know if he leaves,
I will need to confront everything
I have been able to ignore all these years
because he thrust those symptoms upon me
crammed his own opinions in my ears
and I grew deaf to anything else.

It was easy
because I didn't have to face
the confusion,
the raw pain that rippled under my skin

one by one, with every fear that struck
he chased it away and locked it up for me
in a box he keeps in the basement
but the lock can only sustain so much;
if he closes that taxi door
and drives away with his bag of me
of my symptoms,
leaving behind nothing
but a filthy cloud of car exhaust
what will I do in this empty house,
when the lock finally snaps
when all the horrors that are trapped
there finally
escape?

orders

My scale is
a dictator,
a meter that
dictates
whether or not I should be happy.

It measures not my weight
but how much
self-respect and
self-worth
I am allowed at any given moment.

I chose to relinquish freedom of choice
in exchange for the simplicity of doing
without thinking;
for that number quantifies exactly how worthless I am,
which level of punishment
I deserve.

I admit I was enticed by the scale,
its shiny promises and
sparkling numbers.
Only now has it become
dull and faded.

But how can a dictator be overthrown
when its only follower recognizes
its words are toxic
and drinks them anyway
because she loves the way
they taste?

137

How did I reach the point
where everything I am
the way I think
the intelligence I have
my laughter
my relationships
the way I treat others,
the respect I give them
the places I've traveled
my likes
my dislikes
my wit
the things that fuel me with rage
the things that suffocate me with fear
my authenticity
my courage
my humor
the way I process all that surrounds me
my inherent beliefs
my opinions
the wrongs I commit
the rights that make up for them
my worth
has been reduced to
a three-digit number
irrelevant to all of these things?

lake avenue, exit 34C

While I confronted these voices in therapy regularly, I also had to navigate around them on my own outside of therapy. As if they knew I was onto them, the voices only grew more ruthless. They would tell me that I didn't deserve to get better, that my doctors were lying to me about everything, and that I didn't deserve the health or happiness that comes with recovery.

The beginning of this process left me raw and starved for validation. There was no way the voices were going to give me any, so I was left to seek it from another source. I met that source on an online dating app a few months after I began my recovery, and we quickly became attached. He was my first boyfriend, first young love. We made each other laugh, snuggled, and watched TV with a six-pack of beer on rainy Saturday afternoons. I would sometimes catch him sneaking glances at me, because in me, he saw something gorgeous. It was all so mesmerizing.

Soon, my world became all about him. If he wanted to go out, we went out. If he wanted to sleep in, we slept in. I always stayed over at his apartment except for one time when he stayed at mine. We listened to his music, watched his shows. I was an inconsequential part of the relationship.

All that didn't matter. To me, it was never about a partnership between two people, but an exchange; every bit of love my broken soul could give in exchange for the kindness, affection, and external validation I could not achieve on my own. The malicious voices didn't leave but I was able to drown out their pleas with the proof of his admiration of me.

The validation was overwhelmingly addicting, but it was also frail. If he was irritated, I assumed it was my fault. I blamed myself when anything went wrong and always thought I was on the verge of losing him completely. Once while we were baking cookies, I accidentally didn't add as much flour as the recipe called for. He kept mumbling the directions so I couldn't hear him clearly, but I blamed myself for that too. When I saw his disappointed face evaluating the sad state of those cookies, I legitimately thought he might end it right there. Over dilapidated cookies that tasted delicious.

Early recovery is both fragile and hard to quantify. While my boyfriend would support me through this process—such as helping me go to the grocery store without having a panic attack—any doubts I had about our relationship were magnified at every potential misstep.

Unaware at the time, the relationship actually worsened some of the progress I was making in uniting my body and my spirit. I began to use my body as a sort of wall, shielding my soul from further damage. I could engage with him physically, but no way was I going expose my spirit and vulnerability to him. If I let him hold my hand in public or kiss me whenever he wanted to, then I did not have to be completely honest with him about my feelings. An exchange.

While we were together, I was able to ignore all of my own problems because to this one human outside of my core friends and family, I was considered valuable.

✕ ✕ ✕

transitions

At first
when your voice is unfamiliar,
a new being invading my territory

I will love you like a cat.
Guarded, be wary, for
I am very aware of where my claws are,
the number of inches that exist
between my wrath and your porcelain face.

But show affection
and revel in the effects that unfold
as I unfold myself
slowly
to you.

You continue to prove
how safe I am, curled in your arms
until one day I finally seek out the warmth of your lap
all on my own
until I release my trust in a mindful, contented purr.

No longer catty,
I chase you, and
without ever thinking,
without questioning why
I ambush you with affection
because finally, you see,
I love you like a dog.

curls

I love when my hair curls
to match your smile
when you look at me
like I'm a beloved book
and you've just begun your favorite passage
whose words you greedily drink
because every time you let them in
you get to experience their magic
one more time.

worth

I consider my body
a shell for my soul.
I trade my breasts,
my lips
my womanhood
for companionship
as those are the only tokens I have to offer.
To me, the woman inside
is a type of currency
that's no longer accepted here.
Worthless.

waiting

A woman's body
is a mug of hot chocolate;
warm,
cautiously igniting a golden fire
heat gently glowing within you,
smooth,
when you swirl her skin
with your finger.
She is sweet when you first sip her,
letting her beauty cascade over your tongue
yet an aftertaste,
a slight hint of bitter
flickers in her eyes
through her tears
from those times
that they spit in her cup,
added sugar, whipped cream,
for they demanded
extravagance,
divinity, absolute perfection
without first tasting
how delicate
and rich she is,
as she is.
So if she waits
to share herself
until she finds someone with
taste buds so adept to sense
every dimension within
the spectrum of her flavors,
how enticing she is when she stirs,
who can blame her?

dive

My tongue is a diving board
springy and bright, coiled tight.
I often worry my thoughts,
the words
that have been shyly warming up alongside the water
will run
and leap without warning
bounce off my tongue
and splash into the conversation;
though the words may be honest,
they're not ready for a board so high
but my tongue will not discriminate
the words that can from the words that can't—
I often worry that one day
amidst my musings and bad puns
those words will sneak into the arena,
dive the riskiest dive
just to feel the cold rush of the water around them
no matter the consequences that may ensue
those three mischievous words:
I love you

alignment

You embrace me with such tenderness
the billions of pieces of me
collected chaotically
in my body
tug on each other
to arrange themselves
so that I am no longer a puzzle
that someone attempted to build

but abandoned

because something better
came along.

bodily disconnect

I know you mean the best.
I know you like the spirit inside.
I know you don't demand my body.
I know.

I just need you to know that
when I give you my body,
my spirit stays behind.

shielded

The comfort, coziness of a bed
is less so determined
by whether
it beautifully simulates the feeling
of melting
into cumulus clouds
or by how well the mattress
remembers the winding curves of your body;
it is simply more of a matter of
what and who shares the bed with you;

the way they assuage your fears when you squeeze them,
protecting you from the monsters
inevitably hiding underneath.

old orchard road, exit 35

One afternoon, after spending several months accumulating the courage, I handed over my scale—the one tool I used to obsessively quantify my worth—to my doctor. As a scientist and mathematician, I hold the highest respect for numbers, so I would judge myself according to the number on the scale. Numbers were objective. My body dysmorphia may be trying to persuade me that I've gained or lost weight, but I knew how often my brain lied to me about my body. Numbers couldn't lie to me. I saw immense comfort in them. Numbers remained honest no matter how deluded my brain became.

Relinquishing my scale, and therefore relinquishing the numbers that came with it, meant giving up my only quantitative metric for self-evaluation. In a way, this act also granted me freedom from the numbers that the scale displayed. It was the first tangible sign of progress, and I clung to it.

These beautiful, victorious moments were short and infrequent, but when I recognized their presence, they became sacred. Healing is never a parade of constant wins, and I learned early on that even the smallest of successes should be celebrated, even if immediately after the success I did something counter-productive to my recovery.

But I didn't always grant myself the celebration. Sometimes, I would have to practice celebrating myself in group therapy, where the facilitators would encourage us to each share something positive from the week. Other times (and even sometimes now), I would celebrate by writing a little poem to express myself, because I felt like nobody wanted to hear about it. I still struggled reaching out to my friends and family when things were bad, so how was I supposed to share the good stuff too? Eventually I would open up about these moments with my family and friends, and the act of sharing itself was always another victory to be celebrated. My world began to feel a little less dismal once I began noticing and calling out these small moments of progress. I needed that kind of hope.

✕ ✕ ✕

accomplishment #1

On Friday I ate a pop tart.
To anyone else, this would be
a fleeting moment in the day.
Irrelevant, mundane, forgettable.

To them, it was a snack.
They were hungry, so they ate one.
But to me, until that moment,
pop tarts were the forbidden fruit,
this magical food that, once consumed,
would immediately cause me to gain at least a pound.
At least.

I don't know how it works,

but my brain told me it did the calculations
and the math checked out.
So until Friday, I passed pop tarts in every store.
I wanted them, and I'm certain they wanted me,
but my brain,
my ever-so responsible brain,
would remind me about the consequences
of caving into my desires.

I never doubted or questioned it,
how could I?
The math worked out.
But on Friday my belly begged
for a package of pop tarts,
Just one package, it pleaded.

My brain tried say no, but that's when it happened.
My legs shifted me up out of my chair,
my arms slipped into my jacket,
my feet led us out of the building towards the market.

My brain writhed in my skull,
screaming, shrieking,
but my heart told it to shut the fuck up.

If my belly wanted a pop tart,
it was going to get a goddamned pop tart.
Fuck the math.
The math is just a series of symbols.
The math says I can't live the way I want to live.
So fuck the math today.
Fuck my brain today.

With my hands I purchased a strawberry pop tart.
They delicately tore open the package.

The music of the wrapper crinkling delighted my ears.
The soft colors of the familiar pastry soothed my eyes.
My taste buds hugged the sweet flavors of the treat I'd
forgotten
and at last my belly was satisfied,
released from the prison of my brain for just a moment.

But just a moment was all it needed to know
that it was possible to escape.
The war had just begun.

All my brain had now was its precious numbers,
the numbers that chained me up
and forbade me from myself.
These numbers were weapons for so long
I had forgotten they were just shapes on a page,
squiggles, curves, and lines.

Why did they have so much power over me?
How did they shackle me,
control me,
imprison me?
They're just squiggles, curves, and lines.

They can't tell me if I can eat a pop tart or not.
And so I did.
I ate it.
And most importantly—
I enjoyed it.

No guilt, no numbers, no calculations.
Just a sugar rush from eating
a mediocre yet strangely delightful pastry.

On Friday I bought, ate, and enjoyed a pop tart.

On Friday I took a step towards recovery.
But one day, eating a pop tart will be a fleeting moment,
irrelevant, mundane, forgettable.

And will be glorious.

coincidence?

The day I handed my scale over to my physician
the Spanish word-of-the-day on my phone
read: *fuerte.*

Strong.

I chuckled to myself—
damn straight!
If even my phone thinks I have the inner strength,
maybe I actually do.

✕ ✕ ✕

As I became reacquainted with my body as my
own, I looked for ways to create a more positive relation-
ship with it through movement. While I had always loved
going to the gym, running, or playing sports, my physical
fitness had become so entwined with my eating disorder
that all of it became tainted. The voice of my eating dis-
order liked to use exercise as a bargaining chip. ED would
only allow me to have a roll at dinner if I went for a run
that day and burned off the calories to be gained. Exercise

became unhealthy, competitive, and dangerous, especially given that I never gave myself enough nourishment to sustain the exertion.

When my recovery team banned me from heavy exercise, I needed to find other outlets. I started practicing yoga, an exercise I had given up because it didn't always feel like "enough" to satiate ED. Even when I first started, I felt compelled to accompany my practice with another exercise, like going for a long walk, just to please the voice in my head.

However, the more I practiced, the more compassionate I came to be towards my body, and the more comfortable I became with practicing only yoga. No matter how intense or light my practice was, it allowed me to become fully aware and immersed in my body. I realized that healthy exercise doesn't mean I need to sweat through my shirt; healthy exercise is simply moving my body for the sheer joy of movement and the way it clears my mind. My body and mind benefitted just as much from light yoga practices as they did from the heavy ones; the volume of sweat I produced had nothing to do with it.

During this time, I witnessed my body do wonderful things. I felt good and proud of what my body could do. I went from feeling awkward and weak to powering through some really intense poses. Even small stretches or a few deep breaths helped stitch me back together in the places where ED tore through all the seams.

Yoga isn't about competition or ignoring the pain to push through to a goal; it's about energizing each breath to flow through the body and facilitate the bond between body and spirit. It's about small progress and personal growth each day. I reached across the gap between my physical and spiritual bodies, which at first felt like trying to reach over the entire Grand Canyon.

But each practice I reached again, attempting to

bridge the gap between my body and me. Yoga effectively saved our marriage.

✕ ✕ ✕

accomplishment #2

I'm pretty sure
I have a sixth sense
but for cookies.
I can feel their presence through the air waves
hear them calling out to me
their location a mystery only I can solve.

You can hide them,
cram them
into the unlikeliest of cabinets,
those that are forgotten
the ones you think are fake,
just there for the aesthetic,
until one falls open one day
and you wonder how you really did
live there for all those years
and had never known.
The cookies could be there,
masked by mixed aromas of spices nearby
and their image would be pristine in my mind.
No security measures are too strong
to resist my craving, keep me from realizing my binge.
So in one day,
a few hours,
a few minutes,
they are gone.

Lock them up
and I will become a locksmith.
Leave me just a few on a plate
and I will devour them
hunt for the rest
and feast
until no more exist.
It's not a matter of
will power,
nor
self-restraint.
I simply cave in
to the stronger voice inside of me
I cave in
to the foods so long forbidden,
they become that much more addicting.

When I voluntarily
brought cookies into my house,
I was scared.
I thought their lifetime would be short,
that they should say their last words on the way home
but I made them last
for days.
Days.

I never thought I could use an 's' in such a context
but this week I did.
It's only one week
but it's one whole week.

I may always crave, sense cookies wherever I am
a not-so-hidden bond between us
but the days of wild binges on them
are waning

the days of caving to this craving, imprisoned,
to consume every last one
are numbered.

Not yet,
but soon.

finding

I found a small piece of myself yesterday
disheveled,
worn from the fact that I've
refused to wear it all this time.
In a burst some time ago
I had torn it from me,
rejecting that it was mine,
slamming it against the wall
with such intensity,
it pulled a scream from my chest as it left me
and there it fell. There it remained.
I just hope it's not too chipped
and I'm not too broken
to slip it back into its home.
It's felt so drafty
without it.

fuel

I had forgotten
that when I feel full
my brain buzzes happily
because I am not just full of food
but full of the warm energy that reminds me I'm alive,

to have opinions, tell bad jokes,
to giggle at things that aren't funny to anyone else;
to be full is to be able to fully
express

the wispy soul I had hidden, protected
in a secret room
for so long a time
I nearly misplaced the key.

I had forgotten
that my muscles, my heart,
the blood that surges through me,
are not the only parts of me
that require nourishment.

✕ ✕ ✕

When I first started group therapy, it was terrifying to say the least. This was the first time I had to let others (besides my regular therapist) meet the voices in my head. Thankfully, each session was a safe and supported space. While this helped me practice self-compassion, it also allowed others to call me out when I berated myself or when my voices spoke to the group on my behalf. I would not only share my thoughts and emotions, but also all the judgements I held about myself for having those thoughts and emotions. It was the judgements that my therapist and others would challenge, not the thoughts and emotions themselves.

In turn, I would also participate in recognizing others' cruel self-judgements, despite knowing that they were experiencing many of the same thoughts, behaviors, and judgements as me. Even though I was not in their heads, I could acknowledge when they needed self-compassion. The challenge was then applying that kindness to myself.

Every session, we reworked the language used to talk about ourselves to the point where now I naturally rework some of the language on my own.

For years I pretended that I was okay or crazy or somewhere in between, but I rarely allowed myself to speak it aloud. I craved sharing at the very least the name of my disorder with someone so that I wouldn't be alone, because I desperately wanted to be my complete self around another human. My anxious, depressed, disordered self.

Through group therapy, I was able to build a more robust support team around me, squashing some of this loneliness I felt. By practicing vulnerability and overcoming shame in group therapy, I slowly opened up to more of the people I loved about my recovery. My parents were the first I told as they had been so supportive in college and I knew, without a doubt, that I could count on them. I told them about the voices and how they would talk to me. They didn't deeply understand my disease like my peers in group therapy, but they reassured me of their support and love. Sharing with them and allowing them into my journey brought immense relief. Now, when I went grocery shopping and ED was begging me to binge on everything

as soon as I arrived at my apartment, I could call home,
say "I just went shopping and I'm struggling," and without
skipping a beat, they helped me de-escalate the stress.

✕ ✕ ✕

paralysis

The marionette lays
crumpled on the ground
her arms, legs
bent and crooked.
The paint from her smile starts to chip
once it sees the way
her arms, legs
are jerked and directed
by braided
strings; her willpower to move
constricted by strands of twine,
her only power is in the force of tension,
though strong she is soft
and scissors aren't difficult to find.

The marionette has always known where they were
but it didn't remember how to make
her arms, legs
dance on their own—
or rather
she was scared
that without the strings
she could not entertain
she could not be a playful spirit,
chipper and delightful

she was scared that without the strings,
her arms, legs
would sprawl bent and crumpled on the ground
without the slightest idea of how to
pull
herself up without them, with an ingrained fear
of the consequences
of what might happen

if for just a moment she stretches so high
a soft giggle will escape her,
because the clouds are now so close
they tickle.

budget problems

No one is
so emotionally impoverished
her bank of self-compassionate thoughts
vacant and dusty
that
she can't afford
the calories
of the food she loves to eat.

mangoes

Your lips
are mangoes that gush
with sweetness
tumbling down my chin
so that even after you're gone
I can still taste your soft touch
on my tongue.

accomplishment #3

I found a small blue backpack
at a recycling center.
There was something about it that I instantly loved
and I took it home with me.

It's become my friend that's always up for an adventure
from beaches to mountains
to meandering
the twisted labyrinth of new city walls
it loyally hugged my tanned shoulders.

Inside I'd put water, sunscreen, snacks, and beer
wedged between my courage and self-love
tug its drawstring closed
and let it sag on my back
experience after experience.

After some time, I begin replacing the snacks

with my scale.
The bulky corners poke maliciously at my shoulder blades
its mass gathers all the gravity it could muster
such that the fabric of my little backpack
becomes distorted.

Its soft straps
cut my skin.
My pack becomes too heavy.
I remove one beer.
Two.
Three.

I abandon the sunscreen on a beach somewhere
accepting the searing burns that appear.

I pour all my remaining water
into the grass beside me alongside the self-love it was time
to neglect.

I try to shove in a sweater to keep me warm
but the scale hogs every unit of volume
not even a glove could sneak in.

My backpack
starts to fray
the threads attempt to escape with my withering courage;

Dehydrated,
cold,
sunburned,
hungry,
craving nothing but a cold beer,
I have had enough.

It takes several tries
the scale slips from my sweaty hands
the muscles in my arms strain
but I find the power
the energy
to extract it from my pack.

It amazes me how much room there is,
space I forgot even existed.
Lighter,
I can again traverse paths
that were previously daunting,
forbidden.

Lighter, I can pack my old friend with a picnic
and warmly sit atop a hill somewhere
wrapped in the sun,
enjoying a cold beer.

dempster street, exit 37

I was a bundle of nerves curled in my bed. Despite the work I'd been doing, the last few weeks had been tough; instead of becoming healthier, I was relying on my ED behaviors more and more. The harder I fought to gain independence from my disorder, the harder ED fought to maintain control over me. I could feel his resistance in my body, hear his pleads begging for forgiveness. Even the thought of rolling out my yoga mat or eating a full meal had ED roaring with displeasure, loud enough to burst my ear drums. Very few things appeased him.

As if on its own, my body hopped up from the bed, drove to the grocery store, and bought a feast: giant bags of chips, cookies, nearly anything and everything my body craved. As soon as I arrived home, I scarfed it all down while watching TV on my bed, some show I had probably seen a million times before. Alone with my body, I binged up a storm, until self-loathing and a bloated belly eased me into a dull sleep.

Amidst the success I was making toward recovery, there were long periods where I found myself in a murky lake of unclear feelings like this, forcing myself to just exist no matter how uncomfortable I felt. There was nothing to do in this lake. The water was dark, dreadful, and dangerous. I didn't want to be there, but I was also scared to leave; the darkness felt familiar, comforting, because I'd forgotten how to live in its absence.

I would become frustrated with my therapist when she would tell me to sit through my discomfort and explore the shadow that lurked beneath the surface. "Be curious about it," she would say. Sometimes I didn't even want to go to therapy because I didn't want to give myself permission to explore those emotions, let alone allow those emotions to run free. Curiosity killed the cat, didn't it? I wasn't prepared to face that danger. While I knew her solutions were designed to help, they required massive amounts of effort on my part. Sometimes I just didn't feel like exerting that kind of emotional labor.

My ED behaviors would provide me with a numbness, a stray log to cling to in that uncomfortable lake of feelings, until I was ready to confront them again.

✕ ✕ ✕

withdrawn

It's crumpled in blankets
when nobody knows I'm home
except for that spider in the corner of my room
that I'm too scared to kill

when I feel the most valuable contribution
I can make to this world
is to make no contribution
at all.

self-conscious

what do you mean, "hyper-aware of your body"?
she asked.

I twisted the ring on my finger while I spoke;
I can feel it on me.

a question of adequacy

to feel inadequate is to feel
I'm just a mess you'll have to keep cleaning
the dust that refuses to disappear from my bookshelf.

because I am blind
to myself and yet still trying to see
through the chaos that is me
disrupting the order that is you.

to feel inadequate is to play the song
over and over again on repeat:
aren't you better off without me?

✕ ✕ ✕

I have been to four therapists over the years of my
recovery. Each one encouraged me to tolerate my discom-
fort with emotions, but I still hate it. Don't get the wrong
idea—I didn't keep firing them for giving me this advice! I

simply lived in different cities or changed insurance so that unfortunately, consistency was never a guarantee.

Relapse, on the other hand, was irritatingly consistent. Without a doubt relapse happens, but it is how I respond to relapse that moves me forward.

Relapse has worn different faces for me over the years despite the fact that the names of the voices in my head have always remained the same.

Early on, relapse was tough for me to identify because I was still reluctant to change my thoughts and behaviors. My first months of recovery all kind of felt like a relapse because I was only just gaining an astute awareness of how deeply these illnesses intertwined within my mind and the intensity at which mental illness consumed my life. I was still starving myself, still calculating my caloric intake, still going on four-hour-long walks because I ate something ED forbade. Each meal still induced intense debates about what I wanted to eat versus what ED wanted me to eat. The only difference was that now, I could acknowledge which situations triggered these thoughts and behaviors. But I was nowhere near the point where I could actively stop them.

Only months after beginning my road to recovery, I began exhibiting behaviors of bulimia for the first time. With every inch of progress I made, ED fought to push me back a mile. Early recovery seemed undeniably fruitless and barren. I sometimes wonder if my bulimia came out of a need to cope with the weight of this hopelessness.

Every time I relapsed, I would feel so ashamed. Though each relapse truly is a benchmark for progress in itself, each time felt so low, bleak, and insurmountable. The only way to escape was to wade through the discomfort and emotions that floated, surrounding me, and I honestly couldn't do that.

I felt like I was drowning in them instead.

While I didn't have the physical and emotional strength to overcome every relapse, I swam as far as I could until I reached something more tangible or comfortable. It wasn't ideal but at the time, that was all I could do to keep myself moving forward toward recovery.

✕ ✕ ✕

hiding

I always considered it a skill
to be invisible.
Physically present,
mentally unseen.
I worked hard
to craft those masks I used
so that when they saw me
they saw still seas
blanketed in pale sunsets
roses without thorns
a flurry, not a blizzard.

sorry

Sorry I hurt you.
Sorry I lie.
Sorry I leave you alone while you cry.
Sorry I forget.
Sorry I let you down.
Sorry I'm the reason for your frown.
Sorry I'm awkward.

Sorry my jokes aren't funny.
Sorry it's cloudy when you wish it to be sunny.

Sorry I trip.
Sorry I fall.
Sorry you bump me in busy halls.
Sorry I laugh loudly.
Sorry I mumble.
Sorry when I'm hungry you hear my stomach grumble.
Sorry I cough.
Sorry I sneeze.
Sorry I take some exams with ease.
Sorry I smile weird.
Sorry I'm ill.
Sorry I have talents and interesting skills.
Sorry I'm upset.
Sorry I need you.

Sorry I'm a burden—
I really don't mean to.
Sorry I call you.
Sorry I text.
Sorry I take up space—
or something to that effect.

Sorry you hurt me.
Sorry you lie.
Sorry you leave me alone while I cry.
Sorry I am.
Sorry I was.
Sorry I'm sorry just because.

touhy avenue, exit 39

Some days I would just wake up angry. I wanted to eat, I wanted to feel full, I wanted a goddamn pizza! But every single time ED refused, like I was a small child. Can you believe that asshole? I would be livid. Absolute, un-adulterated road rage.

My anger often took the form of pure defiance. Like a hormonal teenager, I would internally scream, "Fuck the rules!" and go against whatever ED wanted me to do. Oh, you don't want me to eat ice cream? Well how about I eat a whole fucking pint of it! You don't want me to eat dinner today?

Fuck. That.

Oftentimes, this anger manifested itself in my writing. I would dig up my journal, grab a pen, and scribble until I felt a dull pain in my wrist. I would push the pen to the paper with such force that you could see the indentation of the words on the other side. This poor, innocent piece of paper became the victim of my rage. While overall inarticulate, my angry writing could at the very least be described as "colorful."

In these bursts of anger, I would repeatedly ask myself: Why me? Why won't these loathsome voices go away? Why can other people eat a meal without wanting to rip their obnoxious brains out of their skulls? Why can other people go on diets and long walks, but for me it's triggering? How come other people can meet up with their friends without a paralyzing fear their friends will want to go out to eat? I was simply unable to accept that this was now my journey, one I definitely did not ask for. I was fucking pissed off, so I threw a petty temper tantrum. In no way was I mature enough to accept my fate and move on.

My therapist encouraged me to dig into these questions, lean into them. I have never been a naturally angry person; even through all the hoops of health insurance and premiums that would mysteriously increase, I would just calmly sigh and imagine how dreamy it would be to live in a country with socialized healthcare. The fact that I was visibly pissed off in recovery was kind of a big deal.

My writing and my therapist's probing helped me realize that my anger was another, albeit unconventional, sign of progress. I wasn't just angry at my predicament—I was livid that I was being influenced by voices who spread terrible rumors about me to myself. I was tired of giving up the driver's seat. I wanted to take charge of my own path and speak with my own voice, not the voice that had spoken on my behalf for so many years.

The anger I felt was a sign that I was not actually drowning like I thought I was. My head was above the water's surface. The fury also helped me see clearly for the first time that I had the potential to overcome my suffering. A power existed within me, so intense it could obliterate these voices—if I could successfully channel it. While these moments were fleeting, they felt really fucking good.

✕ ✕ ✕

cut the crap

I'm unsure of how you got there
wedged in my throat,
a transformer box.
You let some of my words pass
but mold the others
into your own
with the same flavor as mine;

you think I can't tell the difference
when they slide around my taste buds,
except that yours are easier to produce,
your malleable lies, excuses so weak
they spontaneously combust
as soon as they ooze into the air.

My ideas have the integrity of steel
so don't steal them to spin your wheel
of crap
because I'm armed with tall rubber boots and a big ol' mop
and bullshit is easy to wade through.

hello, godzilla

Sometimes
the only thing I can sense
is the bulk of the body
encasing, choking me;
a ghastly monster
clambering through
a quaint little town,
wisps of my spirit

tangled around its fingers.

gems

They say it's lucky
when you're shit on by a bird.
I'm not saying every drop
is a precious stone
but if you get shit on enough
as life has a tendency to do
think of all the carats
you would accumulate
from the flecks of diamond
embedded within each.

frostbite

How is it
that even though
you are always with me
your rules
constantly guiding me,
I still feel alone?

You say you want to help
that you are my friend
but if that were true
wouldn't you light
the fading tinder within me?

You use your blanket to suffocate it
instead of draping the soft wool
over my shoulders.

If you really are my friend
my savior, always with me,
why do I still shiver?

peterson avenue, exit 41B

Before I even knew what was happening, I took an abrupt turn into relapse. It was a normal Saturday afternoon, and I had texted my boyfriend asking if he wanted to watch a show together. An hour later, he was sitting on my bed, looking at me sadly as he spoke his truth: "I just don't think I'll ever love you." And with that, we were over.

I sat, stunned. My mind was reeling. Not only was I losing a friend, but I was reconnecting with a contrived reality I'd been ignoring that had always reverberated deeply within my core: No man would ever love me.

When he left, I called my parents sobbing as if to rid myself of every ounce of water left inside of me. All of the fear that I'd push him away, feeling like I was constantly trying to keep balance on a giant glass ball—it all shattered, just as I knew it would. I was living in Pennsylvania, away from home, and now I was utterly alone. I know it was an emotional injury, but I legitimately felt pain in my body too.

Between heaving breaths, ED kindly reminded me, "*Now, you really are worthless.*"

I could feel myself losing control. ED promised to make me feel better, if I just followed his simple advice. I agreed, and unlocked the cage in which I stored old coping behaviors I previously locked away. Excited to be freed, they all demanded immediate use. I restricted more consistently, stopped attending therapy sessions, frequently engaged in more binge and purge episodes. I became a true puppet of my disorder, giving ED full reign.

$$\times \times \times$$

closure

You were the bandage, the gauze,
that encouraged me to heal,
shielded me from everything
that tried to rip me apart,
shred me into little, unrecognizable pieces.

Now that you're gone,
torn from my skin
I feel the burning,
the yearning.

The salt from my tears stings
as it slithers into the crevices of myself
still an open wound,
yet to completely heal.

Now that you're gone,
a chapter of my life
written in past tense,
I feel exposed.

I wanted to keep you with me

for so much longer than you stayed.
You claim to not fully stick to me, click with me
but the way you would soothe me,
wrap me so snugly in your arms
tells another story entirely.

A story about a charismatic boy and a chaotic girl
who go together like peanut butter and banana
who care about each other
with the strength of coconut skin.

Yet you ripped yourself away
you believed you didn't quite fit, mold to my skin
cling to me as tightly as I clung to you.

You are a bandage prematurely torn,
but wounds can still heal,
skin cells can grow
without the protection of a bandage.

You were lovely while you stayed,
a glimmer of delight and peace
in a dimly lit life.
You will still be lovely and treasured
now that you're gone
a tattoo on my soul
I could never regret

but now it is time for me
to grow unprotected, vulnerable
embrace my scars
and heal with another layer of skin
so sturdy that
the only wounds it will bear
will barely slice through its surface.

✕✕✕

While I was with my boyfriend, distracted into a false sense of security, all of my symptoms worsened. I wasn't in control of my happiness anymore—I had given up all control to him. I didn't bother to take care of myself because he cared for me and that was more than enough. It was easy to accept his affection as enough when everything else at the time felt unbearable. Unloading everything, shoving my well-being into the bucket of his responsibilities, was truly unfair to him. And at the time, I just couldn't see that.

When he left, the void in me filled with all the lies I'd been telling myself that I was okay. I was completely exposed to myself in a way I could no longer ignore. In his absence, the ceasefire in my mind crumbled as ED flung his most wicked and degrading abuse at me. I could no longer hide behind this thin veil of peace I had found with my boyfriend. The fact that I was cared for by a boy gave me ammunition against the voices. Without it, my defense decayed into nothing. The voices could lash at me whenever they pleased, and there was nothing I could do to stop them.

At the time I felt abandoned, but now I see that this moment was critical. While my boyfriend had always done his best to support me, the solution to my problems was never his to give.

Looking back, I realize that we didn't completely work as a couple and I'm absolutely okay with that. He was very right to break it off. There were things we both could have done better, and this is okay.

But in the moment, I was blind to all of that. In the moment, the loss was a catastrophic pothole I wasn't

prepared for, the damage from which made me reconsider
how reckless I'd been ignoring it all.

✕ ✕ ✕

is this why you left?

I will never understand
how you could hold my body in your arms
lift me up to you and hold me close
and yet you lacked the strength
to do the same with my heart.

multidimensional

I think I will continue to be unworthy of love
until my width approaches zero
and I become two dimensional.

an empire falls

Though you broke your ties with me
you weren't the one to break me
your voice was simply loud enough
to shake the shards of me
weakly held together by weary will
and cause my entirety to
collapse.

loving another without loving myself

To love you is to
be water
       while you're a grease fire

a crystal-clear solution
famous for taming flames
       but not yours.

I'm what you think you want, not
       what you need.

Why burn for me
of all the souls
       when I can only intensify you?

Why return to someone broken
       who will continue to let you fall?

Nothing I have can satiate you
       just as nothing you have can satiate me

how can I give you something I don't have myself?

raindrops are tears from a cloud

Raindrops scurrying down the windowpane,
the tear drops meandering down my cheeks
that leak as pain
bursting from the seams of my eyes
pushing to be free.

Rain, too, is a kind of freedom;
a cloud releasing what it can no longer hold
the burden it has carried and
finally allows to fall.
Majestic, drops tumble from the sky
gently scrubbing dirt from the plants they touch
while giving new life to seeds the dirt has kept safe.

The only difference I feel on my skin
between the rain drops from the sky
and the tear drops from my eye
is the concentration of salt
left behind.

be the marble

I didn't realize I was a block of marble
life cracked, chipped
with a hammer and chisel.

I know I require patience
and will revel at my final form

but until then
all I see
are the pieces
crumbling off
        of me

                toward
                        the earth.

my mistake

I handed you my rawness
sharp but sincere
and you slapped me with reasons
to distrust—
not just others
but the value of my
own damn self;
burning with uncertainty
a trace of your impact
a trace of my injury.

alone and whole

I wanted you,
I wanted you so bad
but I sure as hell didn't need you.

The blood surging within me
still reaches
from the tip of my nose to the tip of my toes

the expansion, contraction of my lungs
breathes more life into my smoldering spirit in a whisper

than the air that rushed from your lips,
every time you kissed me.

cicero avenue, exit 41C

True to our European roots, Oktoberfest has become a sort of family tradition over the years. While I was living hundreds of miles away, my parents would drive to Milwaukee every September to visit my brother at school and celebrate the holiday. I even have a video from one year where the three of them are downing a shot-ski that I will treasure for the rest of my life.

Milwaukee was always too far for a weekend trip, but after the breakup, I needed a change of scenery. I bought a ticket home and escaped for a few days. Essentially, we all ended up laughing and cracking jokes at each other for three days straight. The four of us parading around, drinking, eating, and dancing to the music; it was a sight to be seen. Between choking with laughter that weekend, I reminded myself how to breathe.

Afterwards, I returned to Pennsylvania with all the same problems at all the same magnitudes. Nothing had changed, but I guess I didn't expect it to. Still, that small escape gave me what I needed to recharge enough to keep moving forward.

Travel became a major outlet for me during some of the most difficult moments of my recovery. The never-ending bombardment of emotions triggered during my healing left me straight up exhausted. I was sick of all the fucking traffic. I felt so done with everything around me that I would spend time daydreaming about places I wanted to go instead.

I spent a lot of time planning trips—perhaps to avoid actually dealing with recovery. Some of the trips I ended up taking. From New York City all the way to Tirana, Albania.

Many trips I didn't take.

Recovery requires breaks. For me these took the shape of traveling, either visiting friends in other states or flying across an ocean to learn about other cultures. But they can be small breaks too, and most often were. At first, I wasn't well enough to trust myself traveling long distances, so I might spend the afternoon in a park or make the trek out to Target in the next town over. If Depression was at bay, I would invite friends over to cook an elaborate meal and watch a movie.

Regardless of the forms they took, these moments helped me find brief relief in a journey that would literally take me a lifetime. It's important to put effort and soul into the recovery process, but it's just as important to give myself grace and respite as needed. To completely pause, catch a breath, and admire how just how far I've come.

✕ ✕ ✕

traveler's lament

They say home is where the heart is
but what if my heart is no longer whole?
If little chunks broke off
into Saturdays along the seaside,
drifting in the breeze,
buried in forests, whose leaves I still find
tangled in strands of my spirit.
I've watched as rivers, lakes, oceans
welcome me
delicately pulling little pieces towards them in their foamy
waves.

What if home
is no longer a latitude and a longitude?
But a series of footprints,
a trail of hellos and goodbye hugs,
with new embraces,
but also the embraces I've left behind
in my exploration for flavors, ecosystems,
people I've never before experienced.

What if home buzzes
in a worn backpack in the closet of my mind?
Amidst laughter, the way grass smells during summer
sunrises,
amidst the way you say you love me with your warm eyes,
so earthy yet made from the stuff of galaxies.

What if home is somewhere I carry with me
a destination so remote that only time is sufficient to buy a
ticket?
How do I make my way back?

my reaction to crisis

When I'm lost in my own life
at a roundabout with ninety-three different exits
watching my body move through time
but not live,
not enjoy or choose,
this
is when my desire to be lost
in another country,
another culture,
batch of spices
burns so fiercely
it sears the fringes of my soul.

realization from a room with no windows

When nature hugs me, and I am
pelted by
walking among
melting with
the elements
I am most in my element, untouchable.

In my cozy room
protected from
hiding beyond
invisible to
the elements
I am most bent and bruised.

meditation via the cosmos

Ask me
where I go,
when the sun shimmies under
the dark blanket of sky
so old and worn
the sunlight sneaks through
moth holes and gaps of thread
emerging as stars, nebulae,
galaxies that swirl and float
like the milky froth
on the morning cappuccino
I sip on as I slip off
into the rest of the day.

Ask me
what I'm thinking of,
when the contours of my face
are outlined only by the moon;
I smell the dewy grass in which I lay,
for both questions yield one answer:
traversing the labyrinth of streams
coursing through my chaotic musings.

If you ask,
I'll meet you
where your tributary links to mine,
grab your hand,
and pull you on my raft;
we'll float down the river of our collective thoughts
until the sun groggily begins to stir
and roll up its blanket of dark sky,
so the only reminder of the fading cosmos

is the stardust glimmering in our hair.

Let's sail
until we feel the warm sun
nudge us awake and bring our raft to shore
because its rays finally stretched long enough
to meet us at the earth.

the mississippi

To the river I stride
be it high or low tide
where there are no rules
by which to abide

to the river I've cried
when my strength has been tried
against the waves of the river
my defeats collide

cause at the river I hide
for it will never be snide
no matter the bits of my soul
I confide.

ship routing

If every current
flows in the same direction
cascades, fades
onto the same shore,
why does my boat always land
in the sand of an island
thousands of miles away?

My compass points due north
but its magnet seems more attracted
to
colossal protruding icebergs,
to hurricanes and furious waves
than to the magnetic poles of the earth.

But I'll trust it to navigate me
to the crystalline beaches it seeks,
for sometimes there are days
when the sun hogs the entire sky
silky waves tickle my boat
and I laugh and I can contentedly just be.

I believe I will find those glorious shores
but until that day
I will let the sea breeze play
with my hair,
nap while cuddling the blanket of the sun,
and simply
breathe.

foster avenue, exit 42

No matter how far I traveled or how long I could get away, I always returned home. Each time more exhausted than the last. Not just tired from work or school, but from constantly fighting with the voices in my head. In previous relapses I was familiar with a feeling of numbness, but this time I could feel myself cracking.

Beneath the surface, I felt utter despair. Failure. Sadness. I was brimming with tension and boiling over with emotions.

At times, I preferred the numbness. Numbness was simpler. Numbness, I knew how to handle.

But helplessness, loneliness, shame? I had no idea how to quell that storm. Instead of dealing with these emotions, I would skip dinner and watch TV in bed. The hunger distracted me from the explosion occurring in my mind until I could ease myself into sleep.

This type of defense mechanism was not a new phenomenon for me, nor was this problem. For all those years, I was building up a dam to keep my emotions from leaking out, refusing to let them into my headspace. Every once in a while, the pressure would build and emotions would overflow, but most of the time it contained any emotion I dumped into it.

With each relapse, the emotions continued to mount. With each relapse, I tried to maintain the separation between my being and my feelings.

But the pressure against the dam just kept growing. There was no current, nowhere for them to go. They waited for me, building one on top of another, until they threatened to peek over the top of my dam. I had ignored them for so long that when I finally let myself feel anything at all, be it high or low or anything in between, it seemed they were trying to drown me.

Thankfully, my therapist pushed me to dig a little stream from this growing lake of emotions. At first, the built-up emotions gushed from the lake and overwhelmed the tiny stream I had created. They burst in enormous waves that crashed heavily against me.

Every emotion—and there were many—that surged through me just felt like anxiety at first. I mean, I knew simple emotions like happy or sad, but even those could disguise themselves as anxiety or numbness.

My therapist patiently probed me to untangle the kaleidoscope of feelings that presented itself. Where was I sensing the emotion in my body? What felt off? What happened in the timeline leading up to this emotion?

No longer so isolated, the emotions could finally flow into me. Through me.

The lake not only overflowed, but the water acted as a prism, breaking this generic white-light anxiety into an entire spectrum of different emotions that had for so long hidden themselves. Diverse, complex bands of feelings intertwining and mingling this whole time, and all I was ever previously able to see was anxiety.

Apparently, having this diverse spectrum simply signifies that I'm a human, but this was a hard truth to hear amidst the loudness of the emotions themselves. Originally, my only emotion was anxiety; while loud, at least when I heard an emotion coming, I knew which direction to look. It was always anxiety. But now, in my head and in my body, I heard sounds coming from all different directions, all over this emotional spectrum. I tried to silence the loneliness, just to realize that gratitude was loudly beckoning to me, demanding attention. It was a marathon tending to them all, these new children of mine.

Over time I realized that each time I let myself experience an emotion, as consuming as it was, it came and went more quickly than the time before. It needed significantly less attention. Slowly, I began to stop storing my emotions behind the dam I had built and instead opted to feel them one at a time, as they showed themselves. Receiving more and more attention, the emotions quieted themselves and demanded less of my time.

The pressure began to lessen once I tore down that dam. New emotions quickly flowed through this stream I had built for them. I could acknowledge a feeling, and instead of ignoring it, I became curious about it. I explored it. I created a path, a connection, and I let the emotion flow right through me.

✕ ✕ ✕

facade

Depression is
sewing a smile on an empty face,
patching up the holes in your self
so that no one accidentally wanders in and vanishes
into the hollow space beneath your skin.

molasses

My skin is molasses:
Thick.
Heavy.
Sweet and sticky.
My limbs battle the air for movement.
Every inch is a triumph, every inch is a mile.

With my lungs I heave, my heart
drags in the dirt behind me,
a ball and chain.
My hands reach out,
straining to recapture my spirit,
but it starts to flicker
and my molasses hands lose their shape.

My legs melt, sink,
my spirit disappears,
my heart rolls to a stop behind me.

Meanwhile, inside

bombs of frustration explode,
fragment within me,
aiming to pierce my skin,
attempting to liberate my emotion—
but the molasses absorbs them.

My voice tries to climb up my throat,
an amplified shriek,
a shout, a scream.
But the molasses absorbs all sound.

In my mind thoughts swarm around my skull,
whirring around
around
around.

I can't stop them,
they need release,
they need answers,
they need to be freed.

But quickly they revolve,
around
around
around.

The thoughts, my voice, bombs of emotion,
all pulling the molasses, tearing, stretching,
but the molasses does not give.

They all remain trapped, fending for themselves,
wailing, shuddering, whimpering,
admitting defeat, they slowly
collapse to the ground
with my limbs to meet the earth.

I look back to see my heart behind me
trying to release the war inside
but we both know the molasses is too thick.

And so there I sink, bearing the internal battle,
invisible to the world
leaving them wondering what could possibly be wrong.

hide and seek

I'm not good with my feelings.
Sometimes I catch a glance of one
wishing to catch up to me,
to catch up like old friends
but I nosedive headfirst
into the first shrubbery I see to avoid it.

Sometimes they approach from behind
tackling me in an inescapable hug.
Sometimes it's two or three at a time
and I get embarrassed
because I always mix up their names.

I'm a terrible friend to my feelings.

Sometimes they stand in front of me
blocking me from the rest of my day
walls enclosing me in their monotone little world
their gaze nicking my mind
begging me to acknowledge them.
I try to trick them
a magician waving my scarf
to make them disappear.
Abracadabra!
They blink, exchange
confused facial expressions
and chuckle at me
their foolish friend.

Amusement transitions into irritation
tolerating no tricks.
My feelings, enraged,

begin to swell, until
I am pinned against the wall
their inflated forms pressing on my chest
stealing every molecule of oxygen from my lungs
and promising to only give them back

if I stop hiding
if I give them my attention
if I nurture them

because indeed they are my responsibility.
I should know that, I do know that
but to be their mother, their caretaker
would be to admit that they're real
admit that sometimes I draw a smile on my face with a
crayon
that sometimes I have to chain my hands to my body
to refrain from throwing punches
that sometimes interlaced with my laughter is a tearful
melody.
Admit that I am not a one-person band
and even more so, admit that
I do not have the skills to be one.

Maybe it's not so much
that I'm not good with my feelings.
Maybe I'm just not good at needing.

ED's silver linings

While I was lying on the floor
unable to eat more than a spoonful of pasta,
I felt a hand brush the sweaty hairs
off my face.

ED kissed my forehead,
bent down so his warm breath caressed my ear
and whispered in a voice so proud,
"Good, good.
Keep this up and who knows how
stunning, brilliant you will become."

Two weeks later
I developed blood poisoning.
Hospitalized for five days.
Afraid to recover,
to eat food and regain strength
because it would undo all of the suffering endured
to shrink my body,
it would undo the flattery,
my worthiness of the pride in me,
from ED.

flip

Somewhere inside me
in the room where my emotions sleep
there is a broken light switch.
Too lazy and cheap to call an electrician
they tried to fix it themselves.
Tried.
Wires crossed
black plugged into red
the switch flickers
spontaneously, obedient only to randomness
it flips.
ON.
OFF.
The light jars some emotions awake
but not others.
Without warning
I flip.

wilson avenue, exit 43A

I was still living in Pennsylvania, working as an environmental education intern, attempting to maintain some semblance of normalcy. Despite my parents' constant pleas, I refused to move back home.

I got this, I told my parents, *I am in control.* I repeated this lie to myself over and over until one day—exhausted and emotionally worn out—I broke.

Pause.

I've written many drafts of this book, and every single draft my poor editor suggests that I expand on this breaking point because each draft I glance over it as if it was no big deal.

It is, in fact, a very big deal.

It's comical to me; here I wrote an entire book, laying out my whole life and all of the intricacies of my mind, and I could not for the life of me write a sentence or two about this moment of breaking.

Ever since she first suggested it, I rejected the idea so naturally she may as well have hit my knee with one of those little doctor hammers. It took until this final draft to realize that this resistance is due to the face that I still hold a lot of shame and sadness regarding this breaking moment. I'm ashamed I let it get that bad, ashamed I didn't ask for help sooner, ashamed of having problems at all. And I'm sad and scared for the girl I was, the girl who broke.

Reflecting upon that moment welcomed back the weight of that shame and sadness, reminded me about the fear. So I just ignored the moment altogether. But this book is about vulnerability, curiosity. And that I have nothing to feel shame for about my experience or my illnesses. I need to lead by example. And so I will.

Un-pause.

After weeks of pretending I was a physically and mentally healthy person, one night I realized that I absolutely wasn't. Depressed and empty, I began the night with a binge, which had then become habit. Then, as had also become habit, I ended it with a purge. The only difference this night was that I noticed I had purged specks of blood in addition to my binge. Terror shocked my system. I could no longer deny that I was unhealthy, that my disease was just a mildly obnoxious friend. The blood told me the reality I refused to hear: my disease wanted me dead.

I immediately texted my parents asking if I could move back in with them. Without hesitation, and with what I'm sure was a great sigh of relief, they agreed.

The fresh pain of my first breakup, my worsening mental health, and the longing I had for home became the push I needed to seek more intensive support.

I essentially put my life on hold and quit everything the next morning. The job I loved, the friends I made—I left it all. Within the next week, I was home.

✕ ✕ ✕

this is what it's done to me

Often times
my pants size
is more convincing
of my self-worth
than the warm admiration
from those I love.

conflicts when leaving the metaphorical nest

I.
When I was small
you gave me a little floatie device
for when I swam.
Do you remember?
Faded pink, with straps
that draped over my shoulders.
I sat inside while it propped up
my tiny fat arms.
Safe, I could paddle wherever I desired.
I could even play with the big kids.

II.
But slowly I turned into one of the big kids.
I still wore that floatie.
It barely fit, but you insisted.
You wanted me to be safe
and I only wanted to please you
so I wore it contentedly.

I kicked my gangly legs
flailed my arms
moving only a meter or two,
three if I was lucky.
But I never complained
because it made you happy.

III.
Now the floatie can barely keep my arm afloat
yet still you demand that I use it.
Every time I refuse,
you make me feel guilty
for the anguish I'm putting you through—
the terrible choices I'm making.
But I'm done sacrificing
my own desires for exaggerated fears,
done wanting to please you
more than wanting to please myself.
Did it ever occur to you
that I can tread water?
It was you who taught me how to swim—
don't you trust your own teachings?

I do.

IV.
All I want is to swim and explore
without inhibition.
I know you love me
I know you will catch me
when I'm out of breath
but you have to let me reach that point.
Otherwise how will I ever know
how far I can go?
What I can accomplish?

Who I am outside of the world
I saw in my floatie when I was little?
The world is big, yes,
but I'm no longer small.
Your support got me to where I am
and it will get me to where I will go
but when will you realize I'm tall enough
to ride all of the waterslides by myself?
Realize that there are lifeguards who are watching too.
That even in the open seas I'm never alone.

V.
So keep my little pink floatie
for when I'm too tired.
Hold onto it for me
while I snorkel through the ocean.
I can't wait to tell you about the fish I see,
the bright colors of the coral reefs,
the adventures I'll have embarked on
when I return from them.
Because I love you too much
need you too much
to never swim back.

to ED's other lovers

The greatest tragedy
is that our love is overcapacity
yet none spills over
into ourselves

✕ ✕ ✕

Once I settled in at home, I began researching the next step in my recovery—I found a sort of daytime rehab called partial hospitalization (PHP), which is essentially six hours of daily therapy and lunchtime meal support.

I was reluctant to sign up at first; a part of me still thought I wasn't "bad enough" to warrant such intensive treatment. At the same time, I knew it would be the fast track to true recovery. I made some calls and set up a few entrance interviews to see if PHP was right for me.

Everyone was kind and warm and wanted to help, but I remained skeptical. I still didn't want to believe I had let it get this far. Despite my hesitation, every place I called told me PHP was the right level of treatment for me, if not something more intense. On one of those calls, I was walking around the neighborhood while talking. This was normal for me; I took every chance I could to burn calories. The interviewer noticed the white noise of outdoors and called me out for it. She knew exactly why I couldn't take her call sitting down; she'd seen it before. Helpless and caught red-handed, I relented. I submitted myself into a PHP program the next week.

While I had expected to confront my lurking self-hatred in PHP, I soon realized that I had to relinquish all of my independence as well. Eating, drinking, sched-uling my day—I could no longer call the shots on any of it. My schedule and lunches were completely out of my control. Along with the other patients, we were herded around like little sheep; in a way, this kind of structure is what we needed.

Still, letting go of that independence meant admit-ting to myself that I couldn't take care of myself anymore. As a person who very much likes to write her own story, this stung. A lot.

Perhaps the hardest idea to relinquish was that I knew what was best for myself. I couldn't even trust my own instincts because Anxiety, ED, and Depression skewed every decision. When my support would tell me I needed to eat more, I became defensive. Not that they were wrong, but it served as a reminder that I couldn't always trust my own brain. I had to keep telling myself that independence was something I could earn again; my life, I could not.

Allowing myself to be dependent on others for both support and nourishment was a brand-new experience for me and was ultimately what saved me.

I've been lucky to have always had this support available, but I struggled for a long time to tap into it. I only called my parents when I couldn't control myself in the middle of a panic attack, never just to share my general mental health status. I always assumed that everyone has their own stuff to deal with, and I never wanted to add my problems to theirs.

Only recently have I come to terms with the fact that supporting one another is a vital tenant in the caring-for-other-people contract. As long as I'm capable, I love being there for my friends and family when they're struggling, and I know they feel the same way about me.

By opening up to my loved ones about my recovery, I've also built even deeper connections with them. It shows that I trust them, and I want to let them in. And then they feel they can do the same with me. Tapping into my support team continues to be one of the toughest and yet one of the most rewarding aspects of recovery. It's also the reason I've gotten this far.

✕ ✕ ✕

letter to my body #2: Surrender

The more I starve you
the more famished I become,
the more those knives I used to stab you
dig into me.
As much as I yank
and try to cut myself out of you
I will never escape
because I can never be me
without you.
I am only who I am
because you carried me all this way.
I forced you to wade
through thorny brush and hailstorms
to fend for yourself as I unleashed
the wildest of beasts upon you.
I lashed you with words and thoughts
so wicked I never told anyone about them
(and I still haven't).
I abused you.
I still do.
You've become weathered and broken
because of me
but so have I.
I underestimated your strength
and the extent to which I needed you.
I miscalculated how proud I should be
of the fact that
I am only seen
through you.

letter from my body

I remember, years ago
when I was your home,
when I was more than a cheap studio apartment
with a lease you kept trying to break;
back then, I was your home
the chambers created specially for you
the only place in the galaxy—the universe—
where you would always be safe
and always be welcomed back

a place you respected
because I was yours,
only yours.
Every day you came back
tidied me up
cared for me
took what I gave you
to adorn life on the outside
with your energy that glowed
within the walls of my skin.
With my hands you
spilled vibrant music into the house
you massaged my feet
running through the sand at the lakefront
my vocal cords, your harp
you delicately played
to tell the stories your imagination concocted
snuggled in the warmth of my skull.

Do you remember
when my arms were simply tools
to climb as high as you could

through the crooked trees in the yard?
Do you remember
when my stomach was the sacred place
you stashed the foods
that tickled my taste buds most?

I gave you the world
but I also gave you a place to rest
when the world became too much
and ever since it did
I've spent every day
waiting in my open doorway
for you.

montrose avenue, exit 43C

Slowly, the walls I had built were beginning to tumble, but many remained for quite some time. I was still unsure if I could trust myself or trust new people, particularly men. I harbored many doubts from my previous relationship and past experiences, knowing that no other person could fill the gap of confidence I needed to give myself first. I was still hiding behind most of those walls when I met my now-current boyfriend.

At first, I felt uncertain whether we would last, whether he would want to stick around, but I quickly felt that with this particular guy, I could legitimately communicate about sensitive topics. Hell, I even had to tell him about PHP on our very first date since the reason I moved back to Chicago in the first place was to recover. We were at a bar, a couple beers in (I needed the liquid courage), and he listened to every word of my story, unfazed. It almost didn't matter why I came back—I was back in town, so we enjoyed the time together. And then the conversation naturally flowed into other streams of thought. I believe an intense debate regarding creamy versus crunchy peanut butter ensued. I realized that he was someone I wanted to keep around.

From the start, this relationship was vastly different than my last. We felt comfortable asking each other questions and being upfront about our feelings. With my ex, I never dared to confront him about any inner turmoil, and he never asked. I suppose I never asked him either. But when my current boyfriend is hurt or curious, he blatantly tells me. Through practice, I've learned to be frank, too.

We built our relationship, day by day, with a solid foundation that could withstand the obstacles triggered by recovery. It also helped that I was surrounded by an entire support team in Chicago, including my incredible parents. I spent my weekdays focusing on recovery and weeknights resting and healing in the warmth of my family. Each weekend when I visited my boyfriend, I'd grown stronger. All of these pieces were missing before.

As we continued dating, I had to re-train my brain to believe that he wanted to be with me; the outside, the inside, everything. I had to remind myself that he legitimately saw me as a person he wanted to get to know, which was difficult because I still had a protective barrier surrounding me, barring me from emotional and physical intimacy. This barrier was twenty-eight-years in the making, constructed from experience after experience, plastered together, one on top of another. It didn't matter that I had no major trauma because all of the small traumas bonded together were nearly as powerful. It was easier to hide behind it, but I knew I had to come out from hiding eventually.

Deep down I knew he respected me, and we liked each other, but it took so much work and patience from both of us to penetrate through to the center.

That barrier is mostly dismantled now, but every time I revisit this section, that time in my life, I feel this deep sadness. I remember what it was like to feel like I couldn't be a complete woman, as if being a woman was a bad thing. I remember how lonely it felt to dissociate when it came to physical intimacy with men, how much shame I felt. I remember that mistrust I once had of men, of myself.

Sometimes I still feel that shame, but now I can work through it. And most of the time, I choose to honor the things that I want, without fear of being judged. Where most men added to my mental barrier when I wasn't looking, I am so grateful that this one particular man stood by my side and helped me tear off one layer after another.

I used to think dating was something that existed between me and another person, but I'm beginning to realize that connecting with others requires that I first connect with myself.

Since my days in PHP, and since that first date with my boyfriend, I feel like I've also been dating myself. I am getting to know myself and my truth. It's been a rocky start, and we definitely still fight sometimes, but I think I'm starting to fall in love.

I'm not there yet, and we're taking it pretty slow, but—full disclosure—I think we're meant to be.

✕ ✕ ✕

I think I found it

I.
He brought out my laugh—
with him, for him,
the dull shined brilliantly,
I was a moth entranced
to the wild light inside I had never before seen.
This might be love.

II.
Soft and gentle,
internally bursting with zest
he nestled into my soul and called it home;
we spoke the same dialect and
challenged the limits of absurdity.
This might be love.

III.
He emerged only in shadows
but sometimes with me he shared them.
Dark, but not cold;
we kept each other warm.
This might be love.

IV.
He was my rag
to wipe away my problems
kind and sweet,
I laid my stability in his hands
Maybe he cared, maybe he didn't
but when he let me slip
I didn't fracture, I shattered.
This might be love.

V.
You knew I was sick
but stayed with an extended hand
to watch as I was nourished back to myself.
It hasn't always been easy
but you are worth the scrapes and bruises
one minute snuggling on your chest
one goofy conversation
one terrible joke that somehow makes me laugh
until my lungs refuse to cooperate

is worth the sweat and struggle
of mending any wounds
from misunderstandings.

This
truly
is love.

toxicity

Sometimes when I cleanse the calories from my body
I imagine ED's face; his voice is more toxic
than anything else that would have been
inside me.

But ED is still there.

I struggle to discard him.
Even now, I've carved chunks of him out of me
but some shrapnel still remains.
It's obvious, obviously volatile
dangerously shimmering

but I fear what would grow
into those cavities
if I completely let him go
what is left of me
when all that's left
is me?

approach with caution

A black hole resides in my core
consuming that which dares to wander too close
I'm not surprised when you say
you don't see this part of me
black holes are difficult to find
so small yet more massive than a thousand suns
they lie amongst sparkling clouds
and ribbons of stars.

Wade through planets
watch for asteroids orbit
don't get too close
I'm not sure you understand
how dark it will get
once within a black hole's grasp
even light cannot escape.

to date an Irishman

To date an Irishman is to date a brick wall
of ancient stones, tired and weathered,
yet solid despite having endured
the most powerful of nature's forces.
You approach with wonder
because its charm is irresistibly alluring
and you spend your afternoons there,
day after day, because of the way
the stones enrapture you with their stories.

And overtime you walk along the wall
and discover a window
unveiling whole worlds to explore
beyond these opaque borders of stone.
Color bursts through the window, a fiery red perhaps
because to date an Irishman is to fall in love
with fire itself; an undeniable spirit
burning behind the wall of stone.
Once you embrace the fire
it reveals new beauty within the darkness
you previously only felt existed
through the pads of your fingertips
and the vibrating echo in your ears.

To date an Irishman may sometimes require
scaling towering walls of ancient stone
and wading through flickering flame,
but once you reach the top
the view is so devastatingly lovely
you realize you would climb a thousand
a million
more
for just one more peek, a taste,
relishing in the indescribable gratitude that the one
he wants to share this peak with
is you.

a valentine to myself

Roses are red, violets are blue,
I wish one day you would love me too.
The way your eyes sparkle when you're passionate as hell,
your face contorted with concern if you saw that I fell.
You place yourself last in every priority queue,
if a loved one is broken you fix them before you.
You're wise for your age, hell, you passed quantum
mechanics!
Yet trying not to trip sends you into a panic.
You can be friends with anyone, they approach you in
flocks,
if guys treat you like shit, you kick them in their cocks.
Friends call you in tears but hang up with dry eyes,
people do actually like you—it's not just a disguise.
You can make yourself laugh without needing to try,
even when you're not at all drunk or high.
You've traveled the world and take risks with no fear,
even when your direction in life isn't that clear.
You walk on tirelessly, you are who you are,
and you don't give a fuck where others set the bar.
Because you want to be you, a babe inside and out,
a person worth knowing, without any doubt.
So this is why I write this valentine to you,
I just wish one day you would love me too.

irving park road, exit 44A

Everything didn't just suddenly become perfect. The other day, I felt so emotionally weary that I wanted to rip off my entire body so as not to feel such intense anxiety anymore. I couldn't tell what triggered it, but the physical sensations told me I was feeling something. I balled myself up and sobbed alone.

When this used to happen, I'd see no way out, looking to use my unhealthy coping tactics. Now, when I feel overwhelmed with emotions, I force myself to do a short yoga video and re-center. This usually ends up with me on my mat in child's pose, sniffling while a little puddle of tears accumulates beneath me.

Gradually, I am able to focus less on how badly I want to discard my body and all the confusing feelings that come with it.

I breathe in, breathe out. I feel my muscles stretch when I push my toes against the mat. I notice what it feels like to press each fingertip into the mat, and the small sound I hear when I pluck them back up to move onto the next posture.

Though in mild hysterics at the beginning, by the end of the twenty-minute video, I am in a clear headspace, ready to confront what triggered the hysterics in the first place.

Go me, I'm fucking nailing it.

I'm not perfect, not miraculously healed, and I still have moments where I feel particularly vulnerable. Even so, much of my old self is slowly returning, including my interest in creating art. As ED and Anxiety grew over the years, taking over more and more space in life, I ended up shedding many of my interests to make room. Music, drawing, poetry. My brain placed so much emphasis on being the best, rather than on art for the sake of giving life a brighter hue.

"If you're not going to be perfect, practice hours a day," the voices would tell me, *"then don't even try."*

Then Depression joined the party and sucked any remaining joy out of activities I loved. It utterly destroyed creativity and passion. Through recovery, I began to crawl out of that dark hole and rediscover the pleasure in art and imagination I used to have as a kid.

Now, I play piano, guitar, sing, color in mandalas, crochet, knit, write, paint, and I'm currently learning how to draw with pastels. Pastels are a bitch but I'm very excited about the prospect of using them correctly. I want to point out, though—and this is *crucial*—that I am terrible at most of these things. I do them anyway because they're fun and so long as I like doing them, who gives a shit? I'm tired of believing I can't.

There is so much fear in allowing ourselves to be creative, as if we can only make something if it is worthy of an exhibit in a museum. Creativity is a part of what makes us human, what distinguishes us from most other living beings. It's an outlet for emotion, expression, boredom, and in my case, recovery.

✕ ✕ ✕

letter to my body #3: apology

Savage
is the most accurate word I can find
to describe what I have been to you.
I thought you were the monster
when it was really me the entire time,
blind to the fact that
you are not my straight jacket
and I am not your prisoner.
I thought you were my rusty cage
but I failed to realize
you would always leave the door unlocked;
I was only trapped by you because
that's the lie I told myself.
If you were really so cruel
would you have boarded dozens of
planes
buses
boats
& trains
walked thousands of miles
to show me views so fantastical
we nearly forgot to breathe?
If you were really so evil
would you have introduced me
to all of the people that made us
laugh
cry
ache
& love
love not just them
but ourselves?
I'm sorry for the things I said,

the ways I abused you.
I hope you'll forgive me
like you always have, because
I crave nothing more
than to slip myself back into your radiant skin
and be
passionately carried
the rest of my life
by you.

alien

I had always thought
my mistakes made me a monster
my wrongs made me a demon
my imperfections made me an alien

when really
all of those things proved
how perfectly human I actually was.

listening

Sometimes a melody strikes me
with such ferocity it gently pulls
tears from my eyes.
I know not why
but let the drops tumble
until I taste them, warm and salty,

on my lips; music is an old friend
so familiar with every wall, corner,
weathered crack in my soul
that it knows where to find
the emotions I carefully hide
because I don't know how to treat them
when they roam free.
The music finds them and holds them
carefully in its delicate beat
holds them out to me
tries to show me they mean no harm
that to feel is simply feeling
that the emotions are mine to care for
mine to love, mine to acknowledge.
Through the melody I cautiously cusp
one in my hands, let it lick my fingers
brush my heart; it tickles
and through my tears I softly giggle
though once the notes begin to fade
they take with them my courage
to nurture this part of me I so greatly fear;
I tuck the emotions into hiding
until I find another melody
that coaxes them back
into my hands.

✕ ✕ ✕

I've built my new life upon a sturdy foundation.
The illnesses still butt into my life, but my response to
them has shifted. Now, I have the skills to cope with off
days and the support to turn to when I'm unsure how. I am
capable of being kind to myself and giving myself grace.
When I mess up, I try not to be angry at myself for it and

move on.

Sometimes now, a relapse moment can feel empowering. When a particularly dark moment tries to shatter me, I try to learn more about where my unhealthy thoughts and behaviors stem from. Instead of resorting to skipping a meal or purging, I attempt to de-escalate the emotion to a more moderate level. In this new headspace, I can confront the emotion and cope with it rationally, just as I did the other day with my yoga practice.

Typically, I use tricks to help me do this, like squeezing a cold lemon or holding ice cubes in my hands, letting the radical temperature shift stop my brain from spiraling. Or with intention, I make a cup of tea, patiently moving through each step, and then experience the tea using all five of my senses.

One time I was so unbelievably nervous for an exam that I had the urge to binge-eat. I stopped at my boyfriend's apartment on my way to school and let him see the fear and worry twisting my face. Patiently, he listened to me and helped calm me down. I don't remember how he did it, but I can only imagine he made me laugh—that has become his signature move. It's highly effective.

Once I shock myself out of the extremely heightened stress response, I can explore and experience the emotion underneath in a healthy way, maybe through writing or a thoughtful walk.

I'm still on this road to recovery and still seeing several doctors. Sometimes I still resort back to safe, familiar, unhealthy coping behaviors: binge-eating, skipping meals, ignoring friends, ruminating on my faults, and berating myself. But those behaviors become fewer and farther between.

This is okay. I tell my support when I'm struggling, and we work through it together.

✕ ✕ ✕

future tripping

I want to travel everywhere.
Everywhere in space, everywhere in time.

But at the same time, all I want is to be here.
Where I am. In this moment.
Then the next. Then the next.
In this space at this time.

So you see the conflict:
I wish to scatter myself across the universe
to occupy every slice of space, every slice of time,
but only my mind is capable of this kind of adventure.

The rest of me can only explore one moment.
Then the next. Then the next.

I'm slowly learning,
"I want to be in every place, every time, in this moment,"

needs to change to:
"I want to be."

step one towards self-acceptance

I am all that I need.
I am all that I want.
I am all that I love.
Always have, always will.

The only difference now is,
it can go both ways.

I need all that I am.
I want all that I am.
I love all that I am.

Not always have, but,
from now on,
always will.

a goal

Body acceptance
is running through the grass
with no shoes, no socks
blanketed with summer breeze
and the laughter that
charges off your tongue
when you realize
your soul is solely fueled
by sunlight and the blades of grass
when they tickle the soles
beneath your feet.

groove

Let the music pull my limbs, twist
bend my spine to the fluctuating beat
I know not if my pulse matches the rhythm
or if the rhythm matches my pulse
each note a drop of blood
a molecule of oxygen
a surge of electricity coursing between my neurons.

As I lose control of my physical self,
I journey through my soul
splashing in my emotions
dipping my toes in their oscillating waves;
in this world, I need no explanations
I need no logic; music is the explanation
the beat is the logic.

When I invite the music in
let it soak through my skin
reality becomes trivial
and I can truly
finally
harmonize with my
self.

addison street, exit 45A

Here I begin to breathe.

This is it. My exit is close. I can see it maybe ten cars ahead of me.

I've made it this far.

And yet I know my journey continues, albeit slower now than before. Moving at five miles an hour is still movement, still progress. Between victories and reclamations of power, there will be moments of breaking and relapse. That's just what recovery is.

It took a significant amount of time for me to develop this type of perspective. Contrary to my earlier beliefs, people are not weak for needing help. I was not weak for needing help, and neither are you if you do. You do not need to be on the brink of a mental break or self-harm to seek help.

In the process of making this shift in how I think, I realized that getting myself help is not only courageous, but as sensible and routine as going to the doctor for a broken bone. Therapy is essentially a doctor's appointment for my mind. It shouldn't hold more meaning or stigma than that.

The emotions that whirled me through those years are not unique, yet I felt alone in them for a long time.

Society tells us to keep our emotions inside because they're somehow shameful. They are not. That would be like saying having ears or skin or a nose is shameful. Emotions are just another biological part of being human. It's useless to resist nourishing those feelings and, on a grander scale, our mental health. The sooner we give mental health the same care and attention as physical health, the more speed we'll pick up rolling down our own life expressways.

✕ ✕ ✕

connection

As I dance
I shrug into my arms
I step into my legs
I zip up my spine
and slowly begin to sense
that my body
almost
actually fits.

letter to my body #4: Reparations

Home is
where muscles pulse and blood always flows
where I once refused to grow into your fingers
and snuggle into the softness of your skin;
my new favorite blanket kept with me always.

Through you I laugh until our lungs borderline erupt
our arms give hugs and our torso receives them.
I chat about abstract ideas
with the concreteness of your vocal chords.

Friends offer support,
family offers love
and I experience it
as a flushing of your heartbeat
their tenderness on your skin
endorphins zipping through your brain

I offer the world the gift of my spirit
through the gift of my body
a beautiful liaison between
what I see on the outside
and what I see on the inside

our connection can be sporadic
but each day, I reach you more
settling into the home I neglected,
the only home I've ever needed
is you.

if I had to define "joy"

Joy is
air rushing
when laughter shuffles from my lungs
when smiles curve on my lips
instead of my lips
adjusting to mirror the crescent moon
when that moment
becomes the moment
when all the moments I have experienced
and all the moments I will experience
become pleasurably
irrelevant.

when I finally get a glimpse of myself

This morning I washed upon the gritty shore
I've been seeking for so long;
I've forgotten how
I ever floated so far away
without knowing
it would take years
through creeks of tears
wading through fears
to find my way back.

✕✕✕

I'm turning onto my exit now. At times, I didn't even believe it existed; it was always so damn far away.

Cue the elation, the disbelief, the pride. I did it. I am living proof that anyone can reach their own personal destination, whatever and wherever that might be.

Hell, I still want to travel further. I have goals I haven't yet reached. I'm still working with a nutritionist to improve my intuitive eating. I want to eventually get off my anxiety medication. And I know I will reach these goals, because I've reached every other exit before me, every benchmark that has marked my progress so far.

I wrote this book because sharing our stories and learning from each other can be such an effective tool for recovery. I want anyone who needs it to have that tool.

As intimidating as group therapy was at first, listening to other people's experiences and feelings was such a gift to me. Reading poetry, literature, and stories from other survivors made me realize I didn't have fight this disease alone.

I also realize I was fortunate to be surrounded by family, friends, and plenty of professional help. What a luxury that is. This is hard to come by, and I had many privileges that allowed me access to these resources. I want to offer this connection with me to anyone who needs it; anyone who needs someone to listen and understand when life gets shitty.

This narrative, these emotions, are human. The feelings of loneliness and self-hatred, sadness and paralyzing anxiety, are universal.

Hear my story and know that I am with you in your pain and sorrow even if it seems like there's nobody else. Hear my story and know that no matter how heavy the traffic, however stagnant you may seem, you are always moving forward.

No matter how slowly, you will reach the next exit. And then the next one.

✕ ✕ ✕

a poem for a friend

At no more than five-foot-three
clouds wish they could float as high
when you stand, you brush
powdered snow off the peaks in the Himalayas
with a gentle gust of your breath.

You are the moon
though you may feel far away
never forget
you can move oceans.

I don't know how, but
no matter the number of asteroids
that crash into your surface
(and there have been a profound number)
you continue to orbit
as jealousy oozes from rays of sunlight
because they pale in comparison
to the pale light you shed
that illuminates even the darkest
of midnights.

wildflower

My dear, you
are a wildflower
confronting a hurricane.
Battered, shredded,
number of petals dwindling
like your energy to remain rooted
in the earth.
With each leaf it plucks from you
you feel less like the flower you are
and more like the dirt from which you grow,
and you bloom
with devastation, black hopelessness.
My dear, you
sway with grace
even when raindrops fall like daggers.
When the wind bends the floral pasture,
combs through it using a brush with broken bristles
rippling through
ripping through
you survey around you; the daisies, daffodils
you think you flail while others dance
but are blind to the fact that
they are just as ragged
and you are just as beautiful.
Every hurricane has a lifetime,
every hurricane has an edge.
And when it clambers past you in the sky,
I promise you
the hug you receive from the rays of the sun
will have never felt so warm.

hardware

In you, I see a sturdy two-by-four
not because you lumber, no,
you glide with grace, sashay,
because you are the backbone
the instrumental piece
of so many musicals.

Caked in sinusoidal swirls of caulk,
splattered in layers of paint
from dull browns
to the wildest, most unsuspecting of colors,
you have been tested year after year
but refuse to warp,
refuse to break like an old-stripped screw
because not even an eighteen-volt impact drill
can strip you of your strength.

The cast can dance, belt out any notes they please,
because they know they have you
unwavering beneath them.
No matter the hell they put you through every show
no matter how many times they screw you over
wound you with deep gashes of the saw
there you are—unfazed, admired—
the cast, the audience awes
because without you, your resilience,
the show could not go on.

just talk to me

It's okay if you're scared
if your future is pixelated
if your wants and needs smear together.
It's okay to feel
like even the weight of a breath
overwhelms you
sends your mind twisting
through a labyrinth of infinite paths
through doorways
that lead to nightmares,
hazy dreams,
musty rooms
clouded by thoughts
you wish to rarely visit.
It's okay.
I will hold the corners
of your breath;
release it with you
collapse the burden
until it's no longer so heavy.
We will war together
with the most daunting of your demons
because it's okay if fear crawls
through your veins.
Share it with me.
Recruit me as a soldier
instead of leaving me behind
do not carry all of your doubts,
all of your fears and worries and confusion
alone.

home

I pull off the I-94 expressway at Addison.

In about fifteen minutes or so, I will reach the building that has become my new home. I moved out of my parents' house a few years after starting PHP to a beautiful Northside neighborhood of Chicago. This is where I come home to, this is where my journey has led me so far.

But I know that my commute doesn't end here. Addison is my exit for now, and it suits me, but I know that I'll take many more roads ahead and discover new benchmarks, new exit signs.

I'll keep growing and life will keep moving forward.

Once I reach my apartment building, I scour the neighborhood for a parking spot that doesn't require parallel parking—I am awful at parallel parking. You'd think I would suck at it significantly less given that I've been parking in the city for many years, but I don't. Some days I get lucky and easily slide my car up against the curb, though most of the time I end up doing a thirty-point-turn to squeeze my tiny vehicle into a spot.

But once I park, the worst is over. Just a short walk and three flights of stairs later, I get to snuggle and hug my cat—very much against his will—and then snuggle and hug my boyfriend, who is much more receptive to it than my cat.

Maybe I'll have a snack, or perhaps crochet in a sunny patch on the couch until my cat brings over his favorite little ball for me to hurl across the apartment. Maybe my boyfriend and I will attempt to make macarons, and maybe (read: very likely) we will fail. It doesn't matter. The rest of the day, the rest of my life, is mine.

Sometimes I still see ED rearing his ugly head out from the dark corners of my mind. Sometimes Anxiety or Depression will feel so heavy, I can't even imagine leaving the warmth and protection of my bed. But that's okay. They can be unwelcome visitors, but they are no longer my roommates. From time to time, I may nod or greet them, maybe even embrace them as old friends, but I stop short of loving them as I once did.

I'm the one driving my own life this time.

Tomorrow, I'll hop right back on I-94, just like I did today. I will encounter traffic and assholes and towering trucks, impediments of all kinds to my progress, but that won't stop me from driving.

For now, I'll turn off my ignition, click the lock button on my keys until my car beeps, and I'll try not to forget where I parked so that tomorrow I can get right back in.

Tomorrow, I'm going to bump up the tunes and roll the windows down. I know what to expect, and I'm ready to face it.

Tomorrow, I'll shift into drive.

✕ ✕ ✕

look up

Even
when
        you
feel
like
        you
have
fallen
so
far
down
the
infinite
well
that
the
lonely
darkness
nearly
erases
        you

look for my reaching hand above.
Gravity is the weakest of the natural forces and
one we can overcome; so hold
my hand with nuclear strength and watch us rise
no matter how sweaty or dirty or bloody you are
my hand will never slip
because even though you
may never believe it, remember
you are worth saving.

acknowledgements

I cannot even begin to describe how grateful I am and have been for my mom and dad throughout this process. I know they don't think they handled my breakdowns the right way, but I want them to know that they did. What I needed was endless love and they gave it to me without question. This part probably seems long-winded and rambling (for better or for worse, I'm just like my dad in this way...) but thinking about everything my parents have done for me and with me to help me reach this exit of the expressway in my life renders me incapable of forming proper sentences.

I would like to thank my little brother as well for the constant unwavering support. I remember one time in high school when I was having an anxiety attack surrounding my difficult homework assignment and how, on top of that, my protractor was a piece of shit. Riveting, I know. But without questioning me and without really saying anything at all, he took my protractor, made some adjustments, and gave it back working better than ever. This small, wordless act of kindness propelled me through the attack and is just one of many examples of my brother being an absolute baller.

I would like to also thank my friends. They have always looked out for me and been there for me, through my highs and my deepest lows. Thank you for the meandering conversations about topics ranging from human rights to poop jokes. I direct so much love and gratitude to you all.

Thank you to my current boyfriend, R.E.H. I still can't believe I didn't know your real name the first few months we dated. Or that you had dimples. You are a beautiful, patient, goofball of a person and you constantly give me more reasons to love you.

Thank you to my professional support staff, including therapists and nutritionists. I know it's your job to help me and I pay you to do so, but it doesn't negate your prominent roles in my success.

Finally, and I promise this is the last one, thank you to my lovely editor, Lauren Riebs. If you have a writing project in mind, hire her. This story would have been unreadable and significantly less powerful without her careful editing and keen eye for storytelling.

I am just so moved by the ways these individuals have given me the love I needed to finally be able to love myself the same way. Thank you. This success is as much yours as it is mine. I love you all.